MAGNET THERAPY

Balancing Your Body's Energy Flow for Self-Healing

Holger Hannemann

 Sterling Publishing Co., Inc.   New York

Balance is the connection between being and life. It is the infinity of time, which is the power of time. It is the essence of everything, giving everything its essence. It is the connection between beginning and end, which is pointing from Omega to Alpha and from Alpha to Omega.
—Abbé Alphonse Louis Constant (1810–1875)

I want to express my most sincere thanks to Rita Zeller. Working tirelessly, she was instrumental in bringing about this book and in giving Magnet therapy new life.

My work is dedicated to Newport University

Library of Congress Cataloging-in-Publication Data

Hannemann, Holger.
    [Magnet-Therapie. English]
    Magnet therapy : balancing your body's energy flow for self
-healing / by Holger Hannemann.
      p. cm.
    Translation of: Magnet-Therapie.
    Includes index.
    ISBN 0-8069-7378-1
    1. Magnetotherapy—Popular works. 2. Biomagnetism—Popular works.
3. Self-care, Health. I. Title.
    RM893.H2813   1990
    615.8′45—dc20   90-36927
                                                       CIP

English translation by Elisabeth E. Reinersmann

10 9 8 7 6 5

English translation © 1990 by Sterling Publishing Company
387 Park Avenue South, New York, N.Y. 10016
Additional material © 1990 Holger Hannemann
Original edition published under the title *MAGNETTHERAPIE:
Selbstbehandlung* © 1983 by Frech-Verlag, Stuttgart
Distributed in Canada by Sterling Publishing
% Canadian Manda Group, P.O. Box 920, Station U
Toronto, Ontario, Canada M8Z 5P9
Distributed in Great Britain and Europe by Cassell PLC
Villiers House, 41/47 Strand, London WC2N 5JE, England
Distributed in Australia by Capricorn Ltd.
P.O. Box 665, Lane Cove, NSW 2066

Sterling ISBN 0-8069-7378-1 Paper

Contents

Foreword

Many years ago when I began to lecture, teach, and write for the general public about holistic healing, it became clear to me that there was still a great deal of room for development in the area of simple, effective healing methods. And indeed more and more people in need of help are reaching out to the proven healing techniques of the past—such as traditional herbal remedies and homeopathy, as well as acupressure from China and foot-reflexology.

And as we work with natural healing, we discover that the old tried-and-true methods are still effective today and less time consuming than many modern techniques.

In that spirit, and as the result of many years of work with Chinese healing methods, I am presenting in this book a method of healing that encompasses a variety of techniques—segment therapy, acupressure, and magnetism.

Extensive research has been done on magnet therapy in Japan as well as in the West. It has been shown to be extremely effective and a treatment of choice in many hospitals and clinics. Excellent work has been done in America by many scientists and medical professionals, among them Dr. A. Roy, Walter C. Rawles, Albert Roy Davis, and by Professor M. F. Barnothy. They have been able—through extensive and repeated experiments—to prove that magnetic currents positively influence metabolism and support the formation of amino acids (the building blocks for protein) in cells.

In addition, experiments have shown that it is possible to reduce muscle pain due to poor blood circulation or over-exertion. Magnet therapy, therefore, is an effective and safe addition to many holistic treatment modalities and a valuable alternative to acupuncture.

A look at the history of medicine in civilization reveals that the magnet has been used for medical purposes throughout history in different cultures. In China it has been used for thousands of years.

Egyptian documents in hieroglyphics and cuneiform script reveal that magnet therapy was considered an indispensable part of that culture and a valued means of treating diseases. To this day

5

graphic descriptions on walls, columns, and in temples attest to its use. Vast archives containing records of treatments and cures were kept in the so-called "healing temples." Many ancient writers and poets cite examples of this type of treatment.

Plinus, the Roman historian talks about magnet therapy in the treatment of eye diseases, and the French physician Marcel used it to treat headaches. Islamic physician Ibn Sina, also known as Avicenna (980–1037), treated depression with magnet therapy. And, Paracelsus (1493–1541), whose understanding and intellectual genius reached far beyond his time, wrote: "The magnet is the king of all secrets." He used magnets to treat a wide variety of illnesses.

In recent years Dr. W. O. Stark and Dr. P. Kerdaniel analyzed several scientific reports dealing with magnet therapy, among them studies done at the University of Tokyo Medical School. They came up with surprising results: approximately eighty per cent of patients reacted positively to magnet therapy. I have found similar results in my own practice for many years.

This is why magnet therapy is of such special concern to me. In view of the scientific findings and the practical results I have witnessed, I think it is important to bring magnet therapy to the awareness of the interested lay public—particularly to those seeking help.

It is my hope that this book will help to do that.

Prof. Holger Hannemann, M.Sc.
Herisau, Switzerland 1990

Introduction

While the origin of our solar system with its primeval creative power lies hidden in unknown dimensions of time and space, the all-encompassing soul of the universe is a force field that is holding together the entire visible cosmic structure. The mysterious force of this field rules the Universe, as well as the relation between the stars, the earth, and all the planets in its vicinity. Electromagnetic storms taking place about one hundred miles above our blue planet are the result of these energies, which, while invisible, are present in everything that we see.

We humans are exposed to this invisible power from the moment of birth. Every move we make is subject to it. It influences each atom in the human cell, each seed in the center of an apple.

Try to picture this gigantic force field! The human body, composed of five hundred trillion cells with their atoms and molecules, is an energy-laden entity! The forces that govern the body are in perpetual electromagnetic interaction with themselves and with the environment. The survival and well-being of humans, animals, and the plant world are all dependent on this force.

The complexity of the energy process that governs our metabolism surpasses understanding. But we do know that our sensory organs function on very little energy. There is simply no state of health or illness without the participation of the electromagnetic current in our cells.

The oxygen exchange—the primary source of energy that our organism needs in order to support all the vital processes—takes place within the cells. The cell is—simultaneously—matter, energy and wave function. The ongoing electro-energetic process in our bodies has far-reaching significance.

Since every electromagnetic current is potentially a carrier of information it is also possible for bioenergetic intelligence to be transmitted from the environment to the organism. This exchange of information is also taking place within our bodies—a particularly significant point, because that has made possible our evolution from a single cell to *homo sapiens.*

Macrocosm—Microcosm

Over the last two centuries biochemists have made great strides in researching the structure of the cell. But the biological process should not be seen only in terms of its structure. Because to live means to function. Every organ, every cell is directly dependent on and connected with every other part of the body. The holographic system we call "human" has been provided by nature with everything necessary for survival in an ever-changing environment. Hypothetically speaking, one could see this interconnectedness as dependence on a larger system of which ours is only a part, which leads in the end to the whole of the Universe.

This train of thought undoubtedly is the basis for a statement that expresses a fundamental connection: "The universe controlling us is not only around us but within us, within the smallest building block of every cell." The microcosm is the mirror image of the macrocosm.

The Bioenergetic Reservoir of Energy

The human body is a microcosm within a macrocosm and every cell is the product of another cell. In the same way, every daughter cell is a microcosm of the organism in which the transformation from one form of energy to another is taking place; or, to be more specific, where food energy is transformed into biochemical energy. Nature has devised very specific enzymatic processes in order to convert food into substances that the body can use. It is a complex system requiring a controlled flow of electrons within the cell structure.

Speaking of the human cell as a functioning reservoir of biological energy, nobody put it more elegantly than Heraclitus, who said: "Everything flows." Life means flowing!

Antenna to the Cosmos

Much of today's scientific data supports the idea that physical, psychical, and biochemical reactions are a special part of a continuum that has as its essence electromagnetic energy.

In 1923 Soviet biologist Alexander Gurwitsch, who initiated this research, proclaimed, "Every living cell also produces electromagnetical currents." His fellow countryman Georges Lakhovsky, whose work has outlived that of his detractors, was also convinced that the human body and therefore the cells in that body are equipped with biological receivers that react to every stimulus in the environment. He stated: "Every cell in a body is stimulated by the resonating interaction of the rhythmical flow of electromagnetic currents from the cosmos and the environment."

On one hand, these stimuli create electromagnetic impulses within the nucleus of the cell. Within the organism, on the other hand, internal processes—such as the metabolism of food—set electromagnetic cell activity in motion, showing evidence of mitotic genetic radiation. Measurements have shown this to be identical to ultraviolet radiation. The well-known Japanese radiobiologist Hideo Uchida summarized the conclusion of his research as follows: "We can assume with certainty that everything that exists in the cosmos—and therefore life on this earth—is directly influenced by the power of radiation." James C. Maxwell (1831–79) was of the opinion, as stated in his famous "Electromagnetic Light Theory," that this radiation was clearly an electromagnetic phenomenon.

In the 1930s the Italian neurologist Dr. Calligaris also stated: "The human body is equipped with complex systems of contact points—similar to the acupressure points—that serve as a connection to the radiation energy of the Universe." The efficiency of these contact points, their potential and their power, together with the ability of the cells to resonate, determines the well-being of the human organism. It is possible to demonstrate this with the so-called "Kirlian photography" (see Illus. 1).

The examples cited may appear to have broken new ground. But the fact is that the basis for these assumptions is the centuries-old Chinese theory of energy, which I will sketch out in the following pages. Because effective treatment of an ailing organism with magnet therapy does require the understanding of the electromagnetic process.

All holistic treatment modalities have one thing in common with traditional Chinese medicine: They take all the processes of nature into account, believing that there is no strict division between organic and inorganic matter. According to Wilhelm Reich, who discovered Orgone energy, there is a connection between bioenergy (life energy), gravitational energy and Orgon-energy. In a sense, they are all part of the "power of creation." I think they are identical to it. Everything has a common origin and our being is supported and carried on by the whole of the cosmos.

Man: A Bio-cosmic Creature

Every visible and invisible phenomenon in nature is subject to the universal principles of the power of energy transformation. Human beings, as part of the whole, are not exempt from the process. This transformational power, taking place in a continuum of time and space, is part of the cosmic structure and as such corresponds to the creative cosmic purpose. As the fundamental force—with constructive as well as destructive dynamics—it is the giver of life. Man has always stood in awe of this mystery, because in nature the concept of "energy" stands for "natural power." This power is the

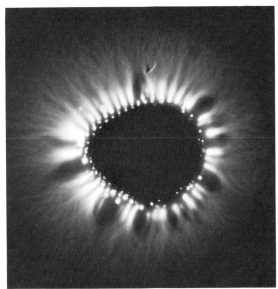

Illus. 1
Kirlian electro-photography, also called "aura photography," shows clearly the "fingertip corona."

guiding, transitive force of evolutionary development. It is present in everything and in all that *is*.

Taoism has given us a symbolic description of the archetypal polarities, YIN and YANG (see Illus. 2), which the Chinese accepted thousands of years ago. It expresses their understanding that every structure in nature, developed according to a higher order, contains two opposing poles, that make up a complete entity. The circle is divided, according to ancient Chinese belief, into YIN, representing the minus polarity and the feminine, and YANG, representing the positive polarity and the male. At the same time, YIN is considered the centripetal (moving in on itself) and passive pole, expressing calm; while YANG is the creative and active force, symbolizing expansive movement.

Both forces reside within every human being. Our organisms—with life force its essential component—obey this natural law. If these creative forces are in balance, we are healthy. Life's energies—in Chinese called "Ch'i," the prime fluid—will be able to circulate freely and consistently through the system and will on a continual basis respond to the environment as well as to the needs of the body.

If, on the other hand, the balance of the energy flow of the YIN-YANG forces is disturbed, the human organism will sooner or later become sick. The loss of balance in the flow of energies or in the

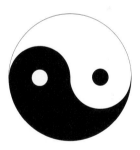

Illus. 2
This ancient Chinese symbol from the Tao depicts both creative forces, the YIN and the YANG. While they are in opposition to each other they also at the same time create each other. The seed of darkness is part of the light; the seed of light is part of the darkness. The dividing line is the symbol of the principle of static and movement. The circle, the all-encompassing Law of the Tao, unites the contradictory pair in the t'ai chi, which is the first beginning that lies beyond every duality.

11

oscillating processes, will diminish activity within the cells and the organism will not be able to function at optimal efficiency.

A Balanced Flow

The body is an indivisible whole. Its balance, being rather fragile, is constantly influenced by the inner and outer environment. The ancient Chinese believe that individual organs influence each other, as they continually strive to support the balance. Therefore, every metabolic activity and the reaction to it is a dynamic process. A living organism is an open system that is constantly expanding but also absorbing energy from its environment and transforming it into biochemical energy. It is this constant exchange of energy that allows the body to maintain its vital balance. So—what appears at first glance to be a static, passive form is actually an organism constantly at work to maintain or regain physiological-biochemical balance.

In this state the body is not only able to transport some of its parts to the surface (such as dying cells and tissues), but it also is able to absorb new substances and convert them into energy. This is most obvious in the processes of nutrition and breathing. In this way, an organism may develop to its highest potential because growth and stability are assured. Should additional energy be needed for any purpose, the process will provide it. There is a flow of give and take in which energy is not lost but made available in a different form. This energy gain is an ongoing creative process and is of vital importance in maintaining good health.

Any interruption in this highly complex energy system would certainly lead to illness were it not for nature's self-regulating and built-in healing capacity, which is always working to bring order back into the system. It is always striving for wholeness.

From this vantage point, it seems clear that if an illness is treated with a narrow therapy, using prescriptions over a long period of time, it will not be able to support this dynamic process. On the contrary, at its worst, it will surely hinder any attempt of the "inner physician" to use the existing self-healing powers.

Energy System and Life Energy

The human energy system is indeed bizarre. It consists of so-called "energy channels" that most likely were established in the embryonic stage. One could compare them with the currents that exist in a magnetic field. These channels, called "Meridians" (see Illus. 3 and 4), circulate life energy through the human body. The meridians transmit the guiding and regulating codes that allow our bodies to maintain a balanced flow of energy. Our health depends on the "organization" of the system. Everything we have been able to learn about existence points to the importance of this "life energy" process. On the one side is a well-organized system that we refer to as health; on the other is illness. To say it another way: life energy must have a coordinated direction, or there is chaos.

In order to better understand this concept, let's compare it to how "Information" is transmitted in a cybernetic system. The information triggers impulses in specific organs, which in turn pass on messages that will effectively guide the energy into a metabolic process, such as creating heat or movement or the like.

This process is not only important for the physiological functioning of the system. It is also responsible for a highly sophisticated mechanism that regulates and keeps in balance the energy flow between the different bodily functions. It influences the breaking down of complex substances, such as protein, into simpler forms; it regulates body temperatures; and it keeps the chemical condition of the blood within rather narrow limits.

In the case of illness, certain points become irritated and the flow of information breaks down. Magnet therapy—much like acupuncture—reestablishes order in the energy household and thereby allows healing to take place.

Why is it that so many different illnesses can be successfully treated with magnet therapy? That is easy to understand when you keep in mind that many illnesses are the result of the same basic dysfunction. Every illness is a bioenergetic breakdown of the organism. It is a sign that the cells have been deprived of energy and the defense mechanism weakened. It is the task of magnet therapy to remove the blockages that get in the way of normal functioning.

1. Magnet Therapy— How It Works

The mysterious power of magnetism fascinates people wherever and whenever they come into contact with it. As mentioned earlier, the discovery of magnetism in China dates back many centuries. In the West, it took a bit longer. Legend has it that in ancient Greece a shepherd named Magnes discovered a magnetic rock. He was leading his sheep across a mountain when the metal tip of his crook entered the magnetic field of the rock. It was only with great effort that he could free the crook. Nobody had a ready explanation, so it was assumed that the rock, which they called "magnet," had a soul. The invisible and unexplained "soul" was the only answer they could find for this unknown and unfathomable power.

It was not until the reign of Queen Elizabeth I of England that William Gilbert (1544–1603) came closer to the secret. His book *De Magnete* contained many fundamental errors, but it was the major work on magnetism until the 19th century. He discovered correctly that a magnet could be divided into smaller pieces without losing its properties. We now know that it is the electrons, circling around the atoms of every iron molecule that create this power.

A magnetic field can also develop through swiftly moving current, as in a storm, or through rapidly changing electrical fields. For instance, a wire ring, exposed to an electrical current, can become magnetized. The wire will show two distinct poles and be able to attract iron. The strength of its magnetic power depends on the amount of electric current applied to the ring.

When this experiment was conducted hundreds of years ago, people did not know that electrical currents were the result of electron activity. The current always moves from the negative to the positive pole. This process is identical to the transmission of an impulse in the nervous system. Chemical, as well as electrical phenomena, are involved in the transmission of an impulse from one part of the body to another. The stimulus of a nerve is described as a self-propelled negative current moving along the surface of the neurons (a unit of nerves). The impulse must have a certain strength in order for excitation to take place. Every active current in the human body creates a small magnetic field.

Measuring devices, developed within the last three hundred years, made it possible to confirm these findings. For instance, Linus C. Pauling received the Nobel Prize in Chemistry in 1954 for his discovery of the magnetic properties of hemoglobin in the blood. This was a significant discovery because iron—in addition to its function as the carrier of oxygen in hemoglobin—plays an important role in the internal metabolism of the cell. Since it is easy to magnetize, iron is a perfect carrier of energy. Here the bonded iron particles in the blood are "lined up," creating an accumulation of energy that—due to its polarization properties (magnetizing of bonded iron and ions in the red blood cells)—strengthens the blood.

A similar change takes place in the property of the water—the fluid of life—in our organism. When magnetized, the surface strength is reduced and molecules, which are lined up in a chain, can separate. This is called a splitting of intermolecular bonds. The result is reactivation of the water household in the organism, which removes blockages and relieves pain.

Magnet therapy therefore has a wide range of application because of its ability to influence the magnetic current in the system. It is always a regenerative holistic therapy, since our bodies are good conductors of magnetic energy.

This conductive property is assisted by the presence of copper in our bodies. This trace element not only helps defend against infection, but it is also involved in the building of red blood cells, the metabolism of pigments, and in supporting the take-up of iron. In addition, copper increases sensitivity to taste and is involved in numerous metabolic processes. It is well known for its support in relieving spasmodic conditions.

Science and Magnet Therapy

Renowned scientists all over the world have been working with magnet therapy. Dr. N. Nakagawa, Chief of Tokyo's Isuzu Hospital, has used magnet therapy on more than 11,000 patients. The primary complaint of these patients was muscle spasm in the shoulder and neck region. For many of the patients, pain was already extending to the upper neck and head and down the back. With magnet therapy he was able to free ninety per cent of the patients from pain.

In another study done in Japan, people were treated exclusively with bio-magnets—these are now available worldwide. Double-blind studies were completed by Dr. S. Arichi at the Hospital of Kinki University and by Dr. J. Suzuki at the Hospital of Tokyo Medical College. They selected 121 patients with severe chronic shoulder pain and divided them randomly into two groups that matched each other in every respect. The treatment of choice was bio-magnets: one group was treated with magnets of a high magnetic strength; the other with low strength magnets. In the active group—with the higher magnetic strength—eighty-two percent showed significant improvement within four days. The control group with lower strength magnets only had a thirty-seven percent improvement rate.

In another double-blind study done in Japan, Dr. Antenucci treated 222 patients suffering from acute and chronic muscle and joint pain (myositis, bursitis, arthritis, rheumatism) with bio-magnets. After only five days ninety percent of the patients in the active group reported lessening of pain, while in the placebo group only fourteen percent reported an improvement.

Extensive experiments with animals at a clinic in Munich showed that wounds and burns treated with magnets were healing very successfully. Numerous experiments with animals and clinical examination of more than 100 patients proved that magnets with static current and those with weaker electromagnetic fields also have a strong influence on the healing process. This was reported at the 91st Congress of the Society of Surgery by Dr. W. D. Mühlbauer, Chief of the Department of Plastic and Reconstructive Surgery at Munich's Technical University.

Another striking success of magnet therapy was reported by a patient who had her abdominal wall surgically tightened. One half of the incision was treated conventionally with sutures; the other half was closed with a so-called "magnetic zipper." After only ten days it was apparent by just visual inspection that the "zippered" portion showed a far greater degree of healing than the other part. The magnetically treated scar also showed the same resistance to tearing. In addition, the formation of collagen fiber in the magnetically treated scar took place in a systematic fashion at right angles to the incision, while the other half showed chaotic, random scar tissue formation.

Good results also have been obtained in the treatment of keloids (hard nodules of fibrous tissue or flattened, streaked skin growth, as in some scar tissue formation). The scar tissue became soft and elasticity was restored.

Similar reports came from Dr. P. Kokoschinegg of the Ludwig-Boltzmann Institute for Acupuncture in Vienna. His greatest success was obtained in the treatment of scar tissue, though treatment time had to be extended. The north pole of the magnets were lined up to the skin of the patients. The magnetic induction was approximately 600 gauss at the center of the pole, meaning it had one thousand times the power of the natural magnetism of the earth. A patient with severe pain and infection after a leg amputation was also successfully treated. He required pain medication at the start, but after several weeks of treatment with bio-magnets, he reported that the pain had disappeared.

Very interesting in contrast is the work that Dr. J. H. Vandyk and Dr. M. H. Helpern from Philadelphia did for the U.S. space program. They raised mice in specially prepared metal cages that shielded them from the electromagnetism of the earth. Within a few weeks the animals lost their fur and began to die. The connective tissue in their skin and internal organs showed signs of uncontrolled growth. Animals raised in a normal environment remained healthy.

These experiments clearly show that magnetic influence varies greatly. But, given the state of today's scientific knowledge, we do not know why positive and negative sides of the magnet can have such diverse physiological effects.

Important in this context: my research shows that the south pole encourages strength and life in all living systems. This means *all* life forms, including invading bacteria, germs, cultures, etc. Therefore, whenever you find any form of infection, use only the north pole—never the south. This is a very special phenomenon of magnet therapy.

Magnet Therapy and the Internal Clock of the Organs

Proper application and treatment with magnet therapy is an empirical science, as are acupuncture and acupressure. When, after the application of a magnetic field, tense muscles relax, blood circulation increases, and the body's own defenses are activated—it is an observable fact. You see at once that magnet therapy is extremely helpful in treating many everyday maladies.

In order to use the negative and positive sides of the magnet correctly we must take into account that the meridians—the

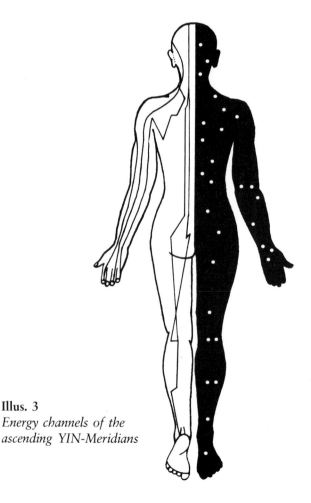

Illus. 3
Energy channels of the ascending YIN-Meridians

energy channels in the human body—also show negative and positive characteristics (See Illus. 3 and 4). The ascending YIN-Meridians have negative characteristics and the descending YANG-Meridians have positive characteristics. The YIN-Meridians proceed from the feet along the insides of the legs to the upper part of the body and down to the fingertips. The YANG-Meridians begin at the fingertips, proceed to the shoulder and head and down to the tips of the toes. Magnet therapy influences the body along the twelve symmetrically organized pairs of meridians that correspond to particular organs—plus the two special meridians that follow the halfway line of the body. Other pain

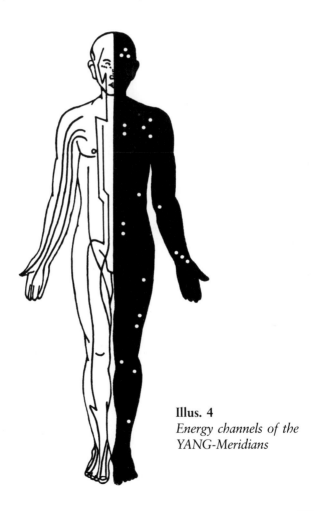

Illus. 4
Energy channels of the
YANG-Meridians

centers, not connected with these energy channels, and some parts of the skin also respond well to magnet therapy.

Various parts of the body and specific pain centers may be treated by the direct application of magnets. But if you're going to treat individual organs, you need to influence them through their corresponding meridians. This is why you need to know about acupressure points and use them precisely. These pressure points are clearly identified in the examples cited in this book. See Chapter 5 for easy-reference charts that identify diagram points and acupressure points that appear in this book.

The effectiveness of both treatment methods may be increased if we take into account the time each individual organ needs for its regenerative process. It is little known that our internal organs operate under a distinct biological rhythm that extends over a twenty-four hour period. Just as high tide is followed by low tide, so do our organs operate at different levels—with each optimum period followed by a recuperation phase. It is important for us to take this into consideration when we schedule our work.

It might seem logical to assume that our organs reach their highest efficiency when we are most active. But this isn't true, as Illus. 5 on page 21 makes clear. Every organ reaches its highest efficiency during a span of two hours. During this period the energy cycle—by way of the meridians—is most active. This has very practical consequences.

The best time for recuperation through sleep begins after 9:00 PM, when the body is recharging its batteries. A further point: Regardless of whether we are sick or well, our bodies should always be in harmony with the magnetic powers of the earth. For this reason, it is best to position the bed so that our heads point towards the north and our feet towards the south. If this rule is followed, the body is in harmony with the magnetic power fields of the earth during the recuperation phase.

We all know that, if a piece of iron is held in a North-South direction and touched by a magnet, it will acquire magnetic powers. And so it is with the human body! This fact is of particular importance in physics, since the alignment results in an energy accumulation that can be compared to a laser beam. A laser beam is created by aligning dispersed energy. The non-aligned energy of a light bulb, for instance, is just about able to illuminate a room, while a laser beam—when its light waves have been aligned—is able to smash through a concrete wall.

To translate this to the human organism, we can conclude that an oversupply of bioenergy will make our bodies susceptible to illness. Bioenergy in balance, however, made possible by a continually flowing interaction between YIN and YANG, will guarantee that the energy potential in our bodies is kept intact.

THE INTERNAL CLOCK OF THE ORGAN

The energy requirements for the organs in our body are subject to a biological rhythm, analogous to the rhythm of the high and low tide. The energy needed for the organs to function is regenerated with maximum efficiency through a flow of energy during the course of a twenty-four-hour day. This schedule is important for the treatment of illnesses, as well as for the intake of medicine. By taking the smallest dose of homeopathic medicine during the optimal time period, an illness can be treated with the best possible results.

Illus. 5   *Optimal Time Table:*

ORGAN/MERIDIAN	ABBREV.	TIME PERIOD	POLARITY	POLE
Liver	LIV	1–3 am	Yin	Minus
Lungs	L	3–5 am	Yin	Minus
Large Intestines	LI	5–7 am	Yang	Plus
Stomach	S	7–9 am	Yang	Plus
Spleen/Pancreas	Sp	9–11 am	Yin	Minus
Heart	H	11–1 pm	Yin	Minus
Small Intestine	SI	1–3 pm	Yang	Plus
Bladder	B	3–5 pm	Yang	Plus
Kidney	K	5–7 pm	Yin	Minus
Pericardium	P	7–9 pm	Yin	Minus
Triple-Burner	TB	9–11 pm	Yang	Plus
Gall Bladder	G	11 pm–1 am	Yang	Plus
Two Special Meridians with regulatory functions				
Conception Vessel	CV	Full-Time day and night	Yin	Minus
Governing Vessel	GV		Yin	Minus

It is extremely important that our bodies—weakened during the day—be remagnetized during the night. The East-West direction is also excellent for a good night's sleep. Here the feet should point west and the head east. The reasoning is that this position is in harmony with the earth's rotation and will help to avoid disturbances that could influence the circulatory system.

The Environment and Its Effect on the Human Body

We have seen that sleep—when the body is properly aligned—is important in the regenerative process, allowing us to relax and recharge our batteries. But in spite of sufficient sleep in the proper position, many people do not feel well when they get up in the morning. Why should that be? During the day we are generally active—at least, we are not stuck in any one place. At night, however, we remain in the same place for hours, and therefore in the same energy field.

Persistent symptoms that manifest in the morning and don't go away—even with good therapy—would suggest that the person is sleeping in a dangerous energy field. The Italian professor Gino Piccardi and the Japanese physician Maki Takata have done research in this area, concentrating specifically on rheumatism and heart diseases. They were able to show a clear correlation between an increased tendency to become ill and exposure to electrical currents. In addition, their research revealed that earth's radiation and magnetic current can alter the chemistry of the blood. Even the functioning of the cell membrane can be temporarily changed. The positive charge of the cell's nucleus and the cell fluid can be strengthened at the expense of the negative charge of the cell's outer membrane.

This shift in the cell's energy field can result in such problems as circulatory difficulties, sleep disorders and an increase in the acidity of the organism. In these cases, external factors, such as stress zones from underground water veins, may diminish our wellbeing and should not be discounted or ignored.

Radiation—a natural part of our environment—is continually being released by disintegrating processes within the earth. This so-called "hard radiation" is everywhere, just as cosmic radiation is saturating the universe. Depending upon the location and its environment—such as the erosion of the surface layer of the ground or the type and composition of the geological formation—hard (terrestrial) radiation can increase in intensity and partially change earth's magnetic field. This means that many people are exposed to the influences of factors, that, under difficult circumstances—a weakened immune system, for example—could threaten their health and wellbeing.

With a good constitution, supported by a biologically natural life style, many people are able to withstand these risks for many years without getting sick. But with advancing age, and when the defense mechanism of the organism is low, the danger of becoming ill increases. This is particularly true during the night, when the influence of the earth's radiation is stronger and the meridians are under constant "bombardment." It is then also that our organism is in a phase of physical, psychological, and mental recuperation, and at its most vulnerable. Sleeping disorders, and anxiety attacks may get started at that time; rheumatic symptoms may appear. Headaches, cramps, congestions of the venous system, may all contribute to these factors.

If we keep in mind that—night after night—the weakest and most vulnerable parts of our organism are significantly burdened by this geopathological stimuli, it is not surprising that so many people living in the same house contract cancer and other chronic diseases that no therapy seems able to cure.

I have seen this situation time and again in my practice. Many physicians report it repeatedly. But to this day no particular attention has been paid to this stimuli as a possible contributing factor to cancer or other chronic diseases. I, for one, do not want to dismiss these possibilities. In the case of those illnesses mentioned above, precautions should be taken: Either the harmful radiation should be eliminated professionally or the bed's position in the room should be changed.

2. Magnet Therapy—Its Practical Application

Physicians in the Middle Ages used clumsy permanent magnets sewn into their patients' clothes, or they tried to mold a magnetic iron to a particular shape of the body. Because of these difficult and unmanageable procedures, magnet therapy fell into disuse. Today magnet therapy has become much more simple and it is again being used as a preferred healing method. Thanks to the development of new alloys, small metal plates of relatively high magnetic power are being manufactured. Japan, for instance, has developed magnets the size of a pea, called bio-magnets, which are sold commercially. They have a barium-ferrite center with a total diameter of only .5 cm (one quarter of an inch). When they are brought into contact with the body, their magnetic flow power is 600 gauss (As a means of comparison: the earth's magnetism has a strength of .5 gauss). These pea-size magnets are attached to a hypoallergenic adhesive support and are very easy to use.

Your skin has to be free of perspiration and impurities before a magnet can be applied. There is no need to remove the magnet when taking a shower or a bath. The alloy will not rust and the adhesive is waterproof.

The optimum effect of the magnet is obtained between the third and fifth day, according to empirical observation. For reasons of hygiene, the bio-magnets should be used only once. If the treatment needs to be continued, use a new magnet. You can double the effectiveness of the magnet if you apply pressure to it—if, for example, acupressure is used simultaneously. According to Professor Bhattacharya and Indian naturopath Samuel Lal, you may also use ordinary magnets that you can purchase in any hardware store.

There are a few important points to consider:

1. The magnets' power and strength (600–2,000 gauss). A guide line as to the approximate gauss power of available commercially sold magnets: Magnets with the lifting power of two

pounds have a gauss energy of 600 gauss. Those with a lifting power of 25 pounds may have a gauss energy of 2,000.

2. The size: They should be easy to handle.
3. Many of the magnets currently available are incorrectly marked.

Don't be confused by the terms "minus" and "plus" or "south" and "north." Both poles have their place in magnet therapy. A deficiency in minus-pole energy in the body, for instance, can block the immune system of an entire organism. So, keep in mind that everything depends on an equal energy distribution for the flow of energy to remain in balance. Bioenergy is constantly circulating, pulsing through our bodies. It is the giver of life!

GOLDEN RULE OF MAGNET THERAPY

The golden rule of magnet therapy is to apply bio-magnets where the pain is—or to use the magnet points indicated on pages 86–87. The bio-magnets take five days to reach full efficiency. Wear them for a week or more. Then pause for two days. If necessary, at that point, apply new magnets and continue the treatment.

The Application of Permanent Magnets

As I mentioned earlier, the Chinese divide the human body—according to the energy channels—into vertical meridians. The front of the body is considered the female YIN (minus) pole and the back of the body the male YANG (plus) pole. When you're using permanent magnets with a pulling power of 25 pounds (2,000 gauss), you need to divide the body horizontally as well as vertically. The horizontal dividing line is the waist and the vertical line is the solar plexus. Vertically, the right side of the body is positive and the left side is negative. Horizontally, the upper part is positive and the lower part is negative. Therefore, in the vertical division, the hands and head are positive, while in the horizontal division, the right hand and foot are positive and the left hand and foot negative. Pay close attention to this segmentation (see Illus. 6–9) because it is the foundation for four basic methods in the application of permanent magnets.

The horizontal division of the body's poles:
Upper part is plus; lower part is minus

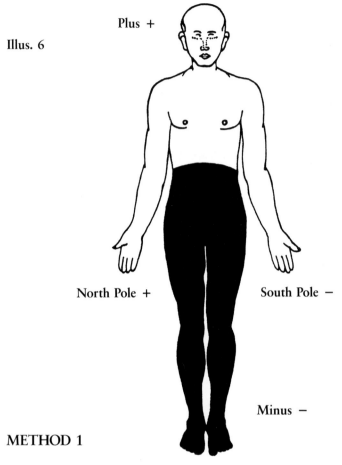

Plus +

Illus. 6

North Pole +   South Pole −

Minus −

METHOD 1

This method is used to activate the kidneys and the urinary tract. In the case of uremia, it can save a life.

For the treatment of uremia attach round permanent magnets—with a pulling power of 25 pounds (2,000 gauss) each—to the sole of each foot. Put the south pole magnet on the left foot and the north pole magnet on the right. For this treatment—as for all others—the patient should be in the North-South position, which means with the head pointing North and the feet South. This treatment is most effective when the timing agrees with the "organ clock"—between 5 and 7 p.m. Leave the magnets on for two hours.

Vertical division of the body's poles:
left side is minus; right side is plus

Plus +

Illus. 7

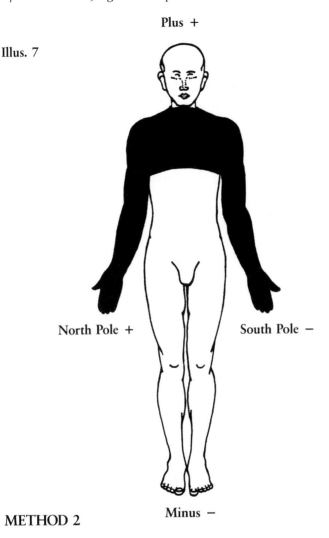

North Pole +   South Pole −

Minus −

METHOD 2

When the problem lies in the upper body—such as tension, inter-costal neuralgia, asthma, or circulatory problems—place one mag-net under each hand—north (plus) pole under the right hand, south (minus) pole under the left. This application closes the circu-lation loop in the upper part of the body. The best time for treat-ment is from 7 to 9 p.m.

27

Plus +

Illus. 8

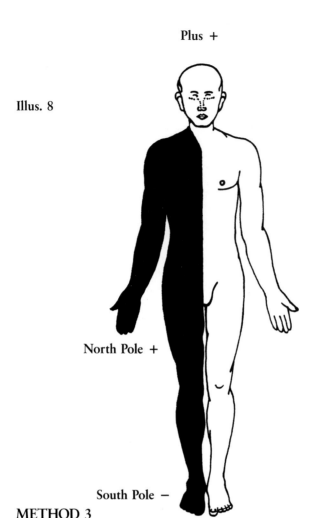

North Pole +

South Pole −

METHOD 3

Minus −

For problems located primarily in the right side of the body, position one magnet's north pole under the right hand and the other magnet's south pole under the right foot. This one-sided application of a strong flow of magnetic current will support the flow of energy to the organs and meridian of the left side. It frees blockages and energy channels. In the case of liver problems and blockages of the portal vein, the most effective time period for the treatment is between 1 and 3 a.m. Additional pressure in the liver area may be particularly helpful.

Plus +

Illus. 9

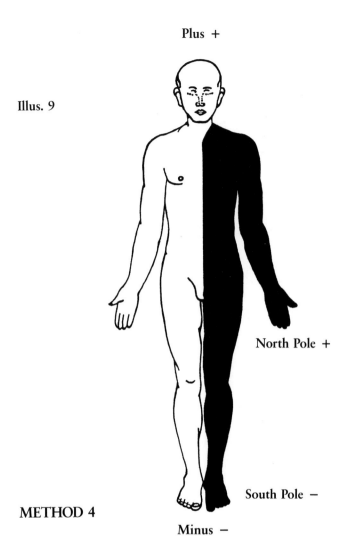

North Pole +

South Pole −

METHOD 4

Minus −

To treat problems located on the left side of the body, apply one magnet to the left hand (north or plus pole) and one to the left foot (south or minus pole).

The Magnet as an Energy Source

If you want to recharge your energy, use Method 1, but add one magnet each under the left and right hands. Put the north (plus) pole under the left hand and the south (minus) pole under the right hand. Altogether, you'll need four Yama magnets. Treatment should not exceed half an hour and is done with the person lying down. It is important that the patient be totally relaxed, breathing deeply and rhythmically with eyes closed. This exercise will help to achieve inner peace. It activates the entire energy household.

Duration of Magnet Therapy

The time allowed for each treatment session depends on the nature of the problem. When you use a strong magnet (2,000 gauss), it will vary from five minutes to two hours. Depending on the patient's progress, you can provide treatment every day—in acute situations, even twice a day. However, when you're using biomagnets you can't follow this system, since their optimum effect is not reached until the third and fifth day. (See the golden rule of magnet therapy, page 25.)

Basic Treatment to Restore and Stabilize Health

It is very important to stick to a well-balanced natural diet that correlates to the season of the year. Only clean food can keep our body clean. Anything in excess and any deprivation can undermine health. Proper, healthy nutrition will give us all the energy our bodies need. The food we eat should include optimal and balanced nutrients and be free of harmful additives, which can burden the system and rob it of its energy.

If, for instance, constipation is a problem, food should contain sufficient fiber to stimulate the peristaltic activity of the intestines. If any form of rheumatism is present, low-acid food is recommended. High acid and denatured food will lead sooner or later to

CONTRA-INDICATION:
WHEN MAGNET THERAPY SHOULD NOT BE USED

As with any other therapy, magnet therapy has its limitations. In case of dangerous infectious diseases, venereal diseases, and conditions requiring surgery, it is best not to use magnet therapy. Although I am not aware of any harm ever having being done with it. I do recommend taking the following precautions, particularly when using strong magnets:

1. People with pacemakers cannot use magnet therapy.
2. Do not attach strong magnets to particularly sensitive parts of the body, such as the heart, the aorta region, or the eyes, neck parts and head regions.
3. Do not use strong magnets during pregnancy.
4. Do not eat or drink half an hour before and after treatment. During the treatment period it is better to refrain from eating food containing meat or animal fat.
5. Finally magnet therapy should not be undertaken with any problem that could potentially lead to complications and should be treated only by medical professionals. When in doubt, check with your physician as to whether magnet therapy is appropriate to use as an adjunct to medical treatment.

a metabolic acidosis, a clogging-up of the entire organism. Metabolism burdened by high acidity will be stressful to the nervous system, and cause tension along with heart and breathing problems, headaches, migraine, gall bladder difficulties, kidney problems, high blood pressure, and much more. For magnet therapy to succeed, it is best to start by breaking the vicious cycle of those problems caused by poor nutrition.

The best way to support the cleansing process is by drinking magnetized water daily. This simple practice is particularly valuable for people suffering from constipation and kidney problems (it assists in the removal of kidney stones). But even without those symptoms, drinking magnetized water is helpful when a general cleansing of the body is necessary. Many studies have shown that magnetized water re-vitalizes the organism.

Finally, it is well-known that almost all enzyme and fermentation processes are possible only within a certain pH-environment. This leads to the following conclusion: Normal metabolism is a physiological process that takes place within the limits of a certain pH value. If the pH-value of your body changes over a prolonged period of time—either to the acid or the base side (you can measure this yourself easily), problems will arise that will considerably influence your health. The acid-base household is continually striving to maintain a balance. This balance, the homeostatis of the organism, is controlled by the autonomic nervous system. But that balance becomes disturbed when the organism has to deal with poor nutrition over a prolonged period of time. Many illnesses result from a disturbance in the acid-base household and the best therapy will avail you nothing, if the nutritional problems are not addressed.

Drinking magnetized water influences not only the autonomic nervous system, but also toxic deposits within the connective tissues. It thereby supports the healing process. Remember, the human body *is* seventy per cent water, and that water is completely renewed every fourteen days. This is why I place so much emphasis on water in the healing process. And this is why using magnetized water is a "basic therapy" for many chronic diseases, particularly where acidosis is at the root of the disease.

PREPARING MAGNETIZED WATER

Preparing magnetized water doesn't take much time. All you need to do is immerse two Yama magnets or one strong magnet (2,000 gauss) with the south-pole side pointing up, under a bottle of water. The magnetizing process takes about ten hours.

Prepare the water at night so that you can begin the next day. Drink half a glass of the water first thing in the morning on an empty stomach. The total daily recommended amount is one liter, which you should drink in four equal portions. Continue the water therapy over several months. (Do *not* refrigerate the water.) This treatment has true energy-building power. It will activate, cleanse, and detoxify every part of the system.

HOW TO IDENTIFY THE POLE OF A MAGNET

While it is important in magnet therapy to use the proper pole of the magnet, not all manufacturers identify the poles on their products, and some identify them incorrectly. Here is a way to solve the problem:

First establish the magnetic needle of the compass by pointing the black side of the magnet needle to the North Pole.

Having established the North-South axis, take your magnet and walk towards the compass. If the needle of the compass turns about 180°, the south pole of your magnet is pointing to the South, and therefore changing the position of the needle. Like poles repel each other! Should the needle of the compass remain in the same direction, the north pole of the magnet is pointing to the compass.

Another way to do it: Using a cylinder type of magnet, tie one end of a thread around the exact center of the magnet and the other end to a high place—the top of a door frame, for example. Allow the magnet to turn. When it stops turning, the end that is pointing to the North Pole of the Earth (use any simple compass to find this direction), is the south pole of the magnet.

Homeopathy Supporting Magnet Therapy

Just as the magnetic field of the earth has a very specific stimulating effect on our bodies, so is the magnet capable of selectively influencing particular organs and tissues. If these organs are in a physiologically susceptible state, they will react quickly to a stimulus that the body would ignore under normal circumstances. Often very subtle stimuli are all that are needed to support life's activities, while the body perceives stronger stimuli as a threat. This has special significance for magnet therapy, which is concerned with the most subtle and delicate stimuli. It usually takes time and patience for the results of the therapy to become apparent. It is therefore advantageous to support magnet therapy with homeopathy, particularly in the case of chronic diseases. The dosage of the homeopathic medicine should be kept low. The body will become tuned to the overall stimuli to a much greater degree when its defense mechanisms and energies are mobilized. The advantage of homeopathic medicine is that the minute stimuli do not add to the disease symptoms, as is the case with allopathic, chemical medication.

Relevant information concerning homeopathic remedies for each condition are suggested under "Additional Measures." In homeopathy the dosage of the medication is geared to the response of the patient, and my suggestions are therefore very general. But the dosages given are within the optimal response range.

GENERAL GUIDELINES FOR TAKING HOMEOPATHIC MEDICINE IN CONNECTION WITH MAGNET THERAPY

Unless I give specific instructions, the general rule is to take ten drops three times daily before a meal with a small amount of magnetized water. Do not swallow immediately. To increase the effectiveness of the remedy, take the drops or tablets half an hour *before* the optimum "organ-clock time" (see Illus. 5). This highly diluted medicine will stimulate energy activity and support the healing process. Keep in mind the cardinal rule of homeopathic medicine: Take only one medication at a time until the desired result has been achieved. Even if there seems to be no reaction, be patient. The body needs a certain amount of time to react to the stimuli, particularly if they are as minute as those applied by the homeopath. In case of a chronic condition, alternate medication with magnet therapy. It is not uncommon in the beginning of treatment for symptoms to get worse. I have noticed this with my patients time and time again. This is a sign that the self-healing energies of the organism are being activated. After the initial phase, reduce the dosage of the medication.

Refer to pages 86–87 for precise placements of magnets for different problems.

3. Treating Illnesses with Magnet Therapy

HEADACHES

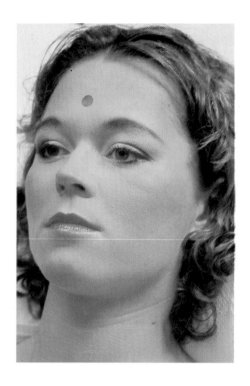

Illus. 10

Vasoconstriction is often the cause of headaches and, while they may be harmless in nature, they may also be a sign of serious trouble. If they persist, it is imperative that the cause be investigated by a physician.

Most of the time, however, headaches are no more than a temporary discomfort. The most common reasons for headaches are tension, alcohol consumption, change in the weather, psychological stress, and the like. These headaches have their origin in the vaso-motor system.

Suggested treatment:

- Acupressure points: Third eye and LI 4
- Corresponding magnet points: 1 and 32

Apply one bio-magnet in the center of the forehead (third eye), plus one magnet each between thumb and index finger on the left and right hands. Repeat application until headaches are gone (7–14 days).

Additional measure:

- Homeopathy: Belladonna D 4, Apis D 4, Gelsemium D 6

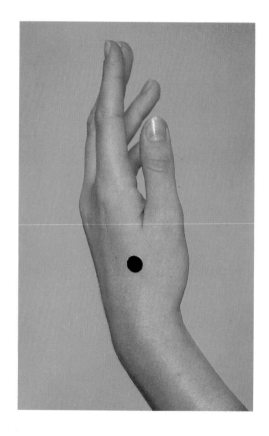

Illus. 11

HEADACHES AT THE FOREHEAD

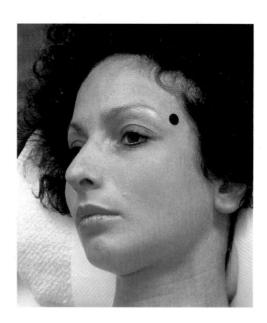

Illus. 12

There is another form of headache where the pain truly is in the center of the forehead, above the eyebrow. These headaches come up suddenly, usually through eyestrain or mental fatigue.

Suggested treatment:

• Acupressure points: TB 21 and LI 4
• Corresponding magnet points: 66 and 32

Apply one bio-magnet each at the indentation located at the end of the eyebrow (TB 21) and between thumb and index finger on both hands (see Illus. 11). Continue treatment until pain subsides.

Additional measures:

• Eye examination by an eye professional
• Kneipp Cure (hydropathic treatment combined with diet and rest)
• Homeopathy: Iris D 3, Belladonna D 4
• Self-hypnosis, meditation

HEADACHES AT THE BASE OF THE SKULL

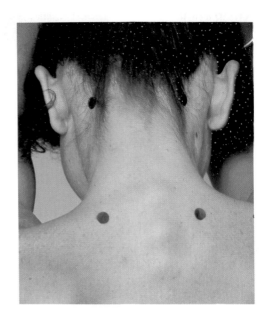

Illus. 13

Pain that is located at the base of the head is usually the result of poor blood circulation due to tensed-up muscles in the shoulder and neck. But the problem might also be caused by a wearing down of the discs of the cerebral vertebra. The latter condition, of course can not be reversed by magnet therapy. But headaches that come from myogenically induced poor circulation can be treated successfully.

Suggested treatment:

• Acupressure points: B 10 and SI 15
• Corresponding magnet points: 16 and 17

Apply two bio-magnets on each side of the cervical vertebra (B 10) at the indentation at the hairline, two additional at the lower cervical vertebra (SI 15) and one at the thoracic vertebra.

Additional measures:

• Exercises: shoulder rolling; lifting and dropping of shoulder; folding hands behind neck and pushing head forward to the chest
• Neck massage
• Homeopathy: Gelsemium D 4, Cocculus D 6

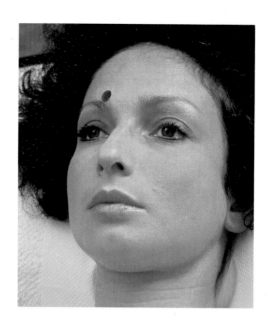

Illus. 14

The onset of migraine headache—when vomiting occurs—is really the endpoint of a chain of preceding problems. Typically, migraine headaches are experienced with piercing pain on one side of the head or face.

Reasons for this pain are manifold and usually result from interference of some sort with the blood circulation in the brain. The cause: Stressful events, such as psychological stress; constipation; lack of sleep; alcohol consumption; anxieties, and tension. In most cases, it takes more than one problem to lead to a migraine attack. It could be the onset of weather turbulence, ongoing constipation, pre-menstrual-syndrome or other related problems, etc. Magnet therapy should be initiated at the first sign of discomfort.

Suggested treatment:

• Acupressure point: B1, L 7 and LI 4
• Corresponding magnet points: 64, 14 and 32

Apply one bio-magnet to the pain site—shown here as above the eyebrow (B 1). Apply second magnet to the base of the wrist at the thumb side (L 7). Place third magnet between thumb and index finger (LI 4, magnet point 32). Continue this treatment for 7–21 days.

Additional measures:

- Shoulder and neck massage
- Suggested elimination or at least cutting back of certain foods, such as strawberries, oranges, mushrooms, tomatoes, eggs, black tea, chocolate, milk, pork and beef.
- Homeopathy: Iris versicolor D 12, Gelsemium D 6, Cocculus D 6, Cyclamen D 4

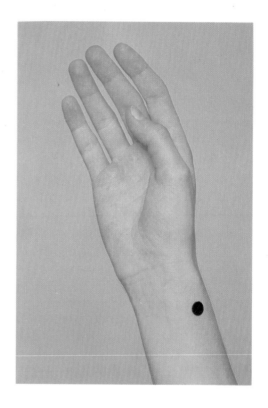

Illus. 15

Additional measures (for Rheumatism, page 41)

- Drinking magnetized water
- Exercising in fresh air
- Eliminating foods with high acid content
- Protection from Earth's harmful radiation
- Homeopathy: Bryonia D4, Colchicum D 12, Dulcamara D 4

RHEUMATISM

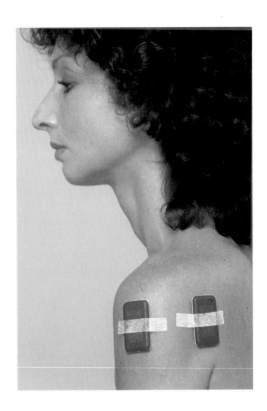

Illus. 16

Aside from any genetic predisposition, rheumatism in its acute stages is often triggered by psychological stress, a cold working environment, sometimes a subterranean water vein (as tension-creating stimuli) in the presence of a toxin-producing metabolic disorder, and by metabolic acidosis, a high concentration of acid in the organism. Infected teeth, tonsils and sinuses may also contribute to the problem. If magnet therapy is to be successful, it is essential that these conditions be treated by a physician first.

Suggested treatment:

Apply two Yama magnets, white side to the skin, or several bio-magnets to the painful region until the pain has subsided (7–21 days).

SCIATICA

Sudden one-sided leg pain (sometimes after exposure to heat), often perceived as a burning sensation, suggests an irritation of the *nervus ischiadicus*—sciatica. The sciatic nerve branches down from the lower back to the thighs and legs. Every one-sided over-exertion of the lumbar region as well as hypothermia or severe strain of the back musculature can cause sciatic problems.

Suggested treatment:

• Acupressure points: B 22, 23, 24, 25 B 50, B 54, B 60
• Corresponding magnet points: 25, 26, 27, 28, 33, 34, 84

In case of an acute attack, immediately apply eight bio-magnets to the left and right side of the lumbar region (B 22, 23, 24, 25), one below the fold of the posterior (B 50), the next one in the center of the back of the knee (B 54) and two additional magnets on the outside between the Achilles tendon and the ankle bone (B 60). The magnets should remain in place at least 8–14 days.

Yama magnets and magnet foil also work successfully here.

Additional measures:

• Move the Yama magnets along the spine, with white side towards the skin, starting from the top down to the feet.
• Drink magnetized water
• Eat food low in acidity
• Homeopathy: Gnaphalium D 4, Colocynthis D 6.

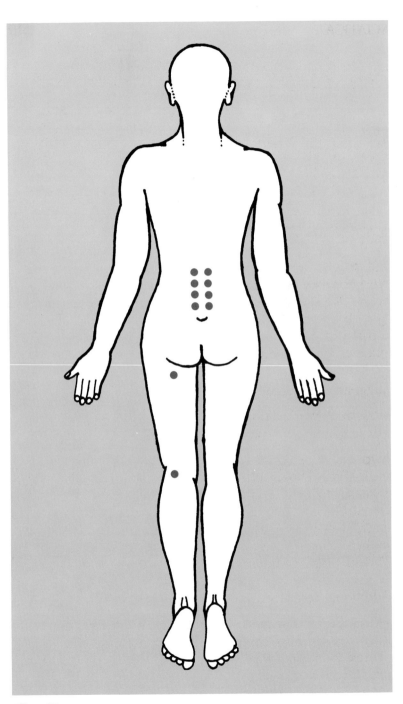

Illus. 17

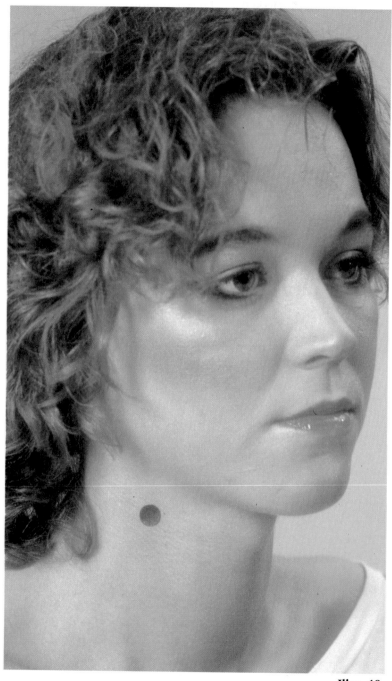

HIGH BLOOD PRESSURE (Hypertension)

Blood pressure is considered high when the level is continually elevated, even after a prolonged rest period. Pressure of 95/160 is considered a limit above which we speak of "high blood pressure." We know that many illnesses have as a side effect elevated blood pressure, one being kidney disease. But high blood pressure is not found only in connection with kidney disease. Metabolic disorders and external toxins like nicotine and alcohol contribute to the problem as well some hormonal imbalances. Anxiety-related stress and psychological stress can also be contributing factors.

Suggested treatment:

• Magnet point: 75

Treatment will be prolonged, even when the pressure is lowered initially. Apply a Yama magnet below the right ear in the region of the aorta, white side facing the skin. Then, using the white side of a Yama magnet, stroke the right underarm, beginning at about half an inch (1.25cm) above the wrist, and ending at the elbow. Do this for fifteen minutes in the evening.

Additional measures:

• Low-salt diet
• Homeopathy: Rauwolfia D 4, Viscum album D2
               If red-flushed face: Aurum D 12
               If pale-faced: Plumbum D 12

LOW BLOOD PRESSURE

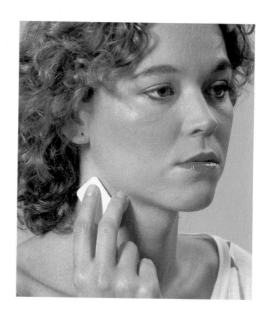

Illus. 19

Low blood pressure is usually accompanied by poor circulation and a weak nervous system. Often psychological, mental and physical stress contribute to the problem. As with high blood pressure, low pressure requires a long treatment period.

Suggested treatment:

Twice daily, for fifteen minutes, apply the black side of a Yama magnet to the region of the aorta below the right ear. During the day also move the Yama magnet, black side against skin, up the entire body beginning at the feet. It is important to check the blood pressure frequently.

Additional measures:

- Kneipp Cure (hydropathic treatment) or alternating hot and cold baths
- Jogging
- Homeopathy: Arnica D 2, Crateagus D 2, Cactus D 4, Kalium carbonicum D 4

SLEEPLESSNESS
(Insomnia)

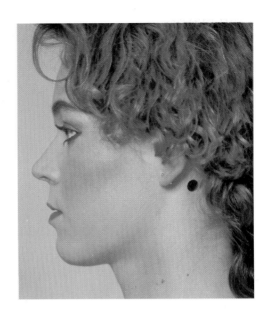

Illus. 20

Difficulty falling asleep; frequent waking up during the night; lack of sleep—each or a combination of all three will lead to depression and a feeling of exhaustion during the day. In eighty per cent of the cases the reasons are psychological, including stress, interpersonal conflicts, worries, metabolic disorders, and the inability to "let go." In later years some people might experience early symptoms of arteriosclerosis and cerebral sclerosis. In these cases, other treatment is in order.

Suggested treatment:

- Acupressure points: third eye and TB 16
- Corresponding magnet points: 1 and 72

Apply a bio-magnet to the center of the forehead (third eye) with an additional magnet at the hairline (TB 16), at a point about three fingers behind the left and right earlobes. Treat for 7–21 days.

Additional measures:

- Self-hypnosis, meditation
- Homeopathy: Zincum valerianicum D 3, Passiflora D 6

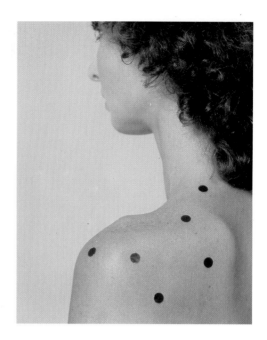

Illus. 21

Muscle tension in the neck region and insomnia are usually the cause of back pain and pain at the base of the head. Habitually carrying weight on one side, one-sided strain on the spinal column, poor posture when sitting, psychological tension; all cause tension. The pain often reaches into the crown of the head.

Suggested treatment:

• Acupressure points: SI 10, 11, 13, 15, TB 15
• Corresponding magnet points: 18, 20, 19, 17, one special magnet point: shoulder blade

Locate the pressure-sensitive points on the shoulder and shoulder blade and apply bio-magnets to them for at least eight days. If necessary, repeat treatment. Also recommended: magnet foil.

Additional measures:

• Neck and shoulder massage
• Exercises: rotating both shoulders, raising and lowering of both
• Homeopathy: Magnesium phosphoricum D 4, Passiflora D 6

LOSS OF MUSCLE TONE (Atrophy of the muscle)

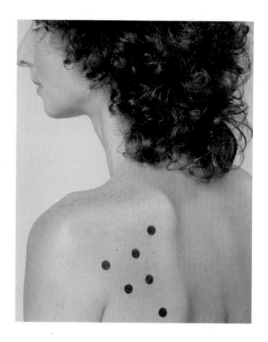

Illus. 22

Reasons for the loss of muscle tone or muscle mass vary. Debilitating illnesses, systemic infections of the spinal cord, lesions of a motor nerve, disuse, insufficient nerve activity of the muscle, and deficient and unbalanced nutrition are some of the reasons for this condition.

Suggested treatment:

Apply several bio-magnets or Yama magnets to the weakened muscle. This increases blood circulation and thereby strengthens the musculature. Treatment should be provided regularly over a prolonged period of time.

Additional measures:

- Movement therapy; muscle-strengthening exercises
- Vitamin E to support protein metabolism for muscle build-up
- Homeopathy: Plumbum D 12, Magnesium phosphoricum D 4

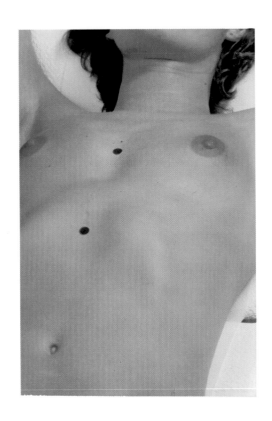

Illus. 23

NEURASTHENIA

Neurasthenia can be a hereditary condition or it may have been acquired. The most common symptoms are mental exhaustion with obsessive behavior, insomnia, and related problems. Unhealthy life style, disturbing experiences, and conflict, as well as misuse of alcohol, nicotine, and drugs may be aggravating factors.

Suggested treatment:

- Acupressure points: CV 15, 17 and S 36
- Corresponding magnet points: 8, 5, 15

Apply two bio-magnets as shown along the sternum, one at the tip of sternum extension (CV 15), and the second in the middle of the sternum (CV 17). Apply two additional magnets to the acupressure point S 36, about 1½ inches apart, two fingerbreadths below the outer edge of the chin. During the night attach an additional magnet to the center of the chin. During the day treat the solar plexus with the black side of a Yama magnet. Treatment will take several months.

Additional measures:

- Breathing exercises
- Drinking magnetized water therapeutically
- Therapeutic herbal health bath with pine needle extract
- Homeopathy: Acidum phosphoricum D 36; Ambra D 4, Kalium phosphoricum D 6, Phosphorus D 4

The sympathetic and the parasympathetic nervous system—two components of the autonomic nervous system—assure the proper functioning of our organs by balanced, reciprocal interaction. The sympathetic system, for instance, increases the heart rate, breathing and pressure in the aortic system, as it slows down the movement and the lymphatic activity of the digestive system. The parasympathetic system, on the other hand, accelerates the digestive process while it allows organs to relax. It slows down breathing and lowers blood pressure, as it stimulates activity and the elimination processes.

With this condition, the balance between the two systems is disturbed. The symptoms are multifaceted and so are the reasons for this state of affairs. Symptoms: Depression, sweaty palms, tightness in the throat, acid stomach, constipation, diminished sex drive, poor blood circulation, dizziness, shortness of breath, constantly being stressed out and in conflict situations. Reasons: Tension at home, stress at work, being overburdened by ongoing interpersonal conflicts. Any of the above will cause the system to dysfunction.

Suggested treatment:

Two bio-magnets applied to the solar plexus as shown will remove the existing imbalance between the two nervous systems. Additional support can be achieved by applying one magnet each to the acupressure points S 36, two fingerbredths below the outer edge of the kneecap. Treatment will take several months.

Additional measures:

• As described for neurasthenia

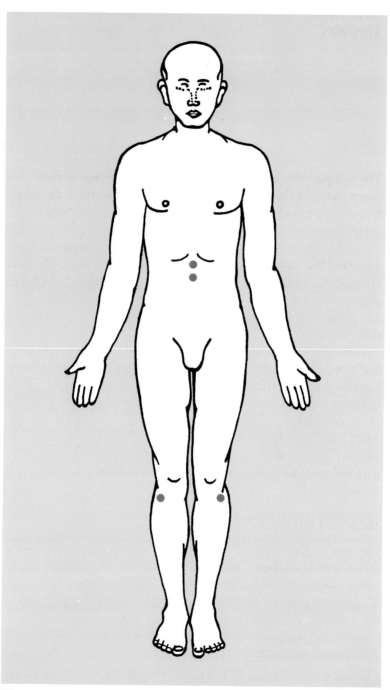

Illus. 24

DISLOCATED ANKLE

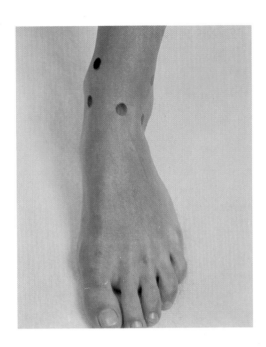

Illus. 25

After a dislocation a careful examination is important to rule out damage to the bone structure. The same holds true for a sprained ankle, which is usually accompanied by bruising. The swelling is best treated with the white side of the Yama magnet. Move the magnet over the whole joint, with special attention to the painful area. Treatment undertaken for fifteen minutes three times a day will quickly bring down the swelling.

Suggested treatment:

Apply bio-magnets all around the ankle as shown for 7–14 days.
• Corresponding magnet points: 56, 57, 59, 84, 85, 87

Additional measures:

• Arnica compresses
• Massage with symphytum ointment
• Homeopathy: Arnica D 4, Symphytum D 2

TENNIS ELBOW

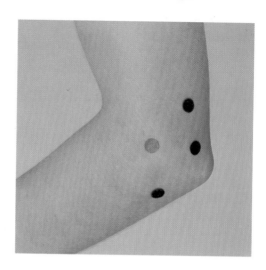

Illus. 26

It isn't necessary to play tennis in order to develop "tennis elbow." Any one-sided motion or over-exertion of the elbow joint could do it. The reason for this problem is a projection at the joint to which the tendon is attached. Faulty playing technique, causing tearing at the site of the muscle-tendon attachment—often leading to inflammation—is usually the reason why tennis players develop this problem.

Suggested treatment:

Surround the painful joint with several bio-magnets. Additional Yama magnet treatment is helpful: Apply two magnets, white side towards the skin, next to each other at the joint. Simultaneously— several times a day for five minutes—treat the area of the shoulder blade and musculature of the back with the black side of the Yama magnet. Continue treatment until the pain has totally subsided.

Additional measures:

• Magnet bandage
• Acupuncture therapy, in chronic cases
• Enzyme therapy
• Homeopathy: Gelsemium D 4

SEXUAL DYSFUNCTION (FRIGIDITY— IMPOTENCE)

One of the most hidden and at the same time most frequent psychosomatic problems is that of sexual dysfunction—impotence in man and frigidity in woman. Both terms are dubious and in no way address the primary cause. In almost all cases, the reason is psychological in nature and directly related not only to sexual issues but to a view of life in general. Psychological blocks, rooted deep in the unconscious, cause disturbances in the autonomic nervous system, which in turn hinder adequate blood circulation and are the cause of weak sexual responses. This in turn brings on tenseness and pelvic tension.

If a real remedy is the goal, it is important first to address the present situation beyond the sexual difficulties—and attempt to deal with the interpersonal relationship between the two partners. At the same time, a strengthening of the nervous system and elimination of the muscle tension is in order.

Suggested treatment:

• Acupressure points: CV 4, 5, Special point "Cli-be"
• Corresponding magnet points: 44, 45, 47

Attach two bio-magnets, as shown, below the navel at the acupressure point CV 4 and CV 5. Next, attach a magnet each at the special points "Cli-be," two energy points at the insides of the thighs. At night, attach Yama magnets to the soles of the feet—one with the black side touching the skin of the left foot and another with the white side touching the skin of the right foot. This arrangement creates a flow of energy throughout the body. Therapy should continue over a long period of time.

Additional measures:

• Herbal therapy with Ginseng
• Vitamin E + lecithin
• Homeopathy: Damiana D 2, Acidum phosphoricum D 3, Muira puama D 4, Zincum metallicum D 8, Yohinbinum D 4

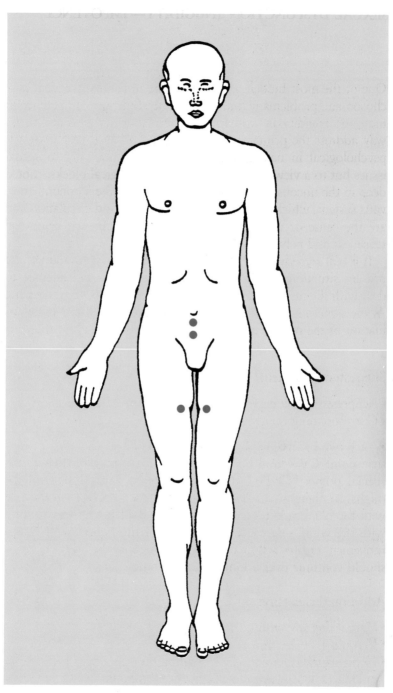

Illus. 27

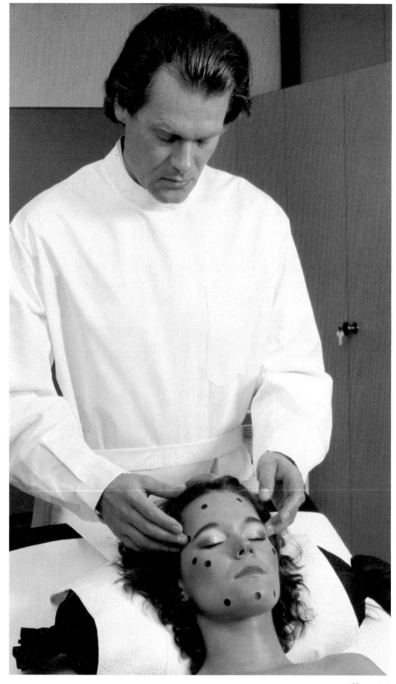

WRINKLES

Small lines give a face expression and life—nobody should be afraid of them! But the deep furrows and facial folds that the poet Tucholsky called the "trenches of life" don't have to be accepted. The fact that magnet therapy is effective for "face-lifting" has surprised many people. After all, face-lifting has been almost exclusively the domain of the plastic surgeon. But a daily regimen of Yama magnets on face and neck will improve blood circulation in the skin, which in turn tightens the facial musculature, and gives the face a younger look.

Suggested treatment:

Gently move a Yama magnet, black side touching the skin, across the face for fifteen minutes like this: From the center of the face outward to the ears; from the forehead down to the ears; from the chin up towards the ears. For even greater strengthening of the facial muscles, apply bio-magnets to the skin as shown in Illus. 31. It is important to be relaxed during this treatment, so lie down while the bio-magnets are applied. Drinking magnetized water will lend further support to the treatment. Wash the face with magnetized water twice daily.

Additional measures:

- Color therapy (violet)
- Jojoba oil
- Therapy with multi-vitamins
- Meditation
- Vocal exercises: several times a day, say aloud: "A, E, I, O, U"
- Homeopathy: Zincum metallicum D 8, Silicea D 4

BLADDER INFECTION Cystitis

Cystitis is a problem that women generally have to contend with rather than men. The ureter being so much shorter in females, it presents a more opportune entry point for bacteria into the bladder. In addition, the wearing of tight panty hose interferes with proper blood circulation in the genital area, which promotes the growth of bacteria. This poor circulation diminishes the body's own defense mechanism, which would be mobilized in case of an infection. Underwear made from man-made fibers also contributes to the problem because of its inability to absorb perspiration. This causes chills, a major factor in acute cystitis.

Suggested treatment:

• Acupressure points: B 26, 27, 28, 58
• Corresponding magnet points: 29, 30, 31, 36

Apply three bio-magnets each to both sides of the sacrum as shown (B 26, 27, 28). Place two additional magnets (B 58) on each calf as shown. The magnets will improve blood circulation in the pelvic area in 14–21 days. Using two magnet foils on the front of the body has also been successful (see Illus. 48).

Additional measures:

• Enzyme therapy
• Therapeutic sitz bath
• Drinking of 1½ liters of magnetized water (lukewarm)
• Bladder and kidney strengthening herbal tea
• Underwear made from natural fiber
• Homeopathy: Cantharis D 12, Mercurius corrosivus D 6, Echinacea D 2

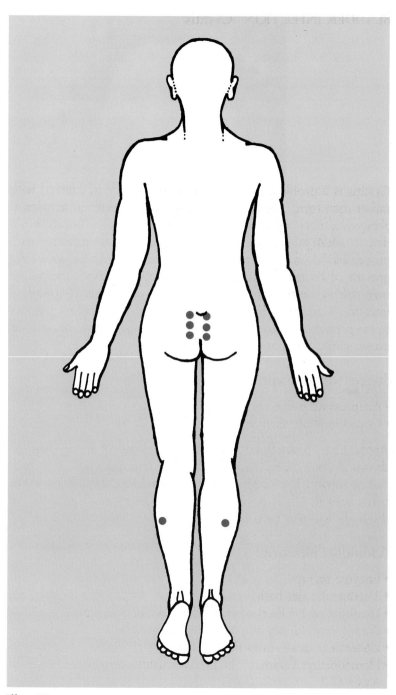

Illus. 29

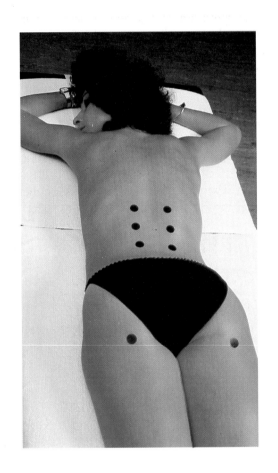

Illus. 30

Backache is not usually the symptom of a serious illness, but it does reveal that the psyche is playing a disastrous role. Tensed-up muscles can cause it, often resulting in unbearable pain in the lumbar region. Poor posture, working in a sitting position, and depression are contributing factors. Women have always had more problems than men with aching backs: on the one hand, a woman's spine has the same resilience as a man's, but on the other, it must be flexible enough to be able to give birth. Most of the time the pain is located within a 6-inch zone (15cm) in the upper part of the lumbar region. If, on the other hand, the pain is more diffuse and in the lower region (the abdominal area), the uterus or the ovaries might be affected and a gynecological examination is called for.

Suggested treatment:

• Acupressure points: B 23, 24, 25, 50
• Corresponding magnet points: 26, 27, 28, 33

Attach three bio-magnets to each side of the spine (B 23, 24, 25) and add two more to the back of the thighs at their highest point (B 50). Treat for 7–14 days.

Additional measures:

• Back exercise (Back roll)
• Back magnet band (belt)
• Yoga
• Therapeutic Bath with the herb rosemary
• Vitamin E + magnesium
• Homeopathy: Gnaphalium D 2, Gelsemium D 4, Nux/vomica, D 4

CONSTIPATION

The nutrients in the food that we eat daily, such as protein, fat, carbohydrates, vitamins, and minerals, become available to our system when broken down by enzymes. Much of our food, however, is denatured; chemicals are added to make it "metabolism-friendly" again and to extend its shelf life. Constipation is usually the result of this one-sided process. Approximately thirty percent of the male and fifty percent of the female population suffers from this condition. Constipation is a sign of sluggish intestines, a condition that is aggravated by a sendentary life style, at home and at work. Matters are made worse by a diet low in fiber content, which cannot support the peristaltic action of the intestines.

Suggested treatment:

• Acupressure points: CV 6, K 15, Liv 13
• Corresponding magnet points: 11, 10, 9

The most important points to treat are above the navel and below the rib cage. They will increase peristaltic activity. Attach bio-magnets to these five points (CV 6, K 15, Liv 13). In addition, give these points a circling massage several times during the day to increase the effectiveness of the magnets. Treat for 14–21 days.

Additional measures:

• Drinking magnetized water
• High fiber diet
• Add wheatgerm to the diet
• Enzyme therapy
• Homeopathy: Nux vomica D 4, Chelidonium D 4, Bryonia D 4, Magnesium chloratum D 4

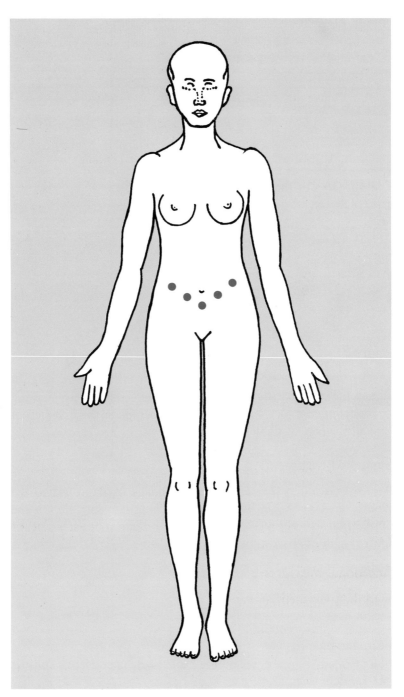

Illus. 31

SORE THROAT

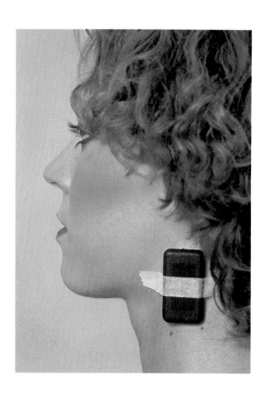

Illus. 32

A sore throat is usually a sign of a tonsil infection with a swelling of the lymphatic pharynx. Use magnet therapy at the first sign of difficulty when swallowing food.

Suggested treatment:

Attach two Yama magnets with a bandage or Band-Aid to the painful area as shown, white side touching the skin. Repeat the application several times during the day for one hour each time, or until symptoms have subsided.

• Magnet point: 75

Additional measures:

• Gargle with camomile
• Enzyme therapy
• Homeopathy: In the beginning Apis D 3, later Hepar sulfuris D 12, Echinacea D 4

HEMORRHOIDS

Aggravated by a sedentary life style and a diet high in animal fat, hemorrhoids are veins in the sphincter that fill with stagnant blood and are surrounded by painful swollen tissue. The patient usually experiences itching and feels the presence of a foreign object. Bleeding, either on the outside or inside of the muscle, is frequently due to infection and this makes regular elimination quite difficult.

Suggested treatment:

First apply a Yama magnet to reduce pain. Attach the magnet, white side touching the skin, above the coccyx (at the end of the vertebral column beyond the sacrum). Leave it on for several hours each day, reducing the amount of time when improvement is noticed. Now and then massage this area with the black side of the Yama magnet. Magnet therapy is very effective here, because it strengthens and tightens the blood vessels.

Additional measures:

- Cod-liver oil will always bring quick relief in the beginning phase. Apply a thin coating to the hemorrhoids during the night. Continue for 2 weeks.
- Suppository made from the extract of horse chestnut
- Therapeutic sitz bath in oak tree bark
- Drink magnetized water
- Homeopathy: Acidum nitricum D 6, Hamalis D 6, Nux vomica D 4

BRONCHITIS

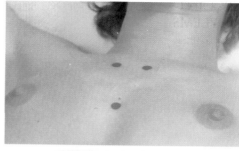

Illus. 33

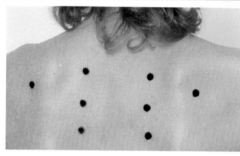

Illus. 34

We know that acute bronchitis involves the swelling of the mucous tissue of the bronchial tubes. At the same time, the body's defenses are diminished; the cleansing process of the cilium does not work well. Dust particles in the air can't be ejected and the damaged breathing passages become narrower due to accumulated phlegm, which in turn causes the alveoli of the lungs to close up.

Suggested treatment:

• Acupressure points: K 27, CV 17, B 11, 12, 13, SI 11
• Corresponding magnet points: 39, 5, 21, 20, 79

Attach two bio-magnets at the edge of the collar bone (K 27), and one magnet to the center at the sternum (CV 17). In addition, attach four magnets each to both sides of the spinal column (B 11, 12, 13) and shoulder blade (SI 11). Treat for 7–21 days.

Additional measures:

• Enzyme therapy
• Homeopathy—In the beginning: Aconit D 30; later: Belladonna D 6, Ipecacuanha D 6.

HIP-JOINT PROBLEMS
(Arthrosis)

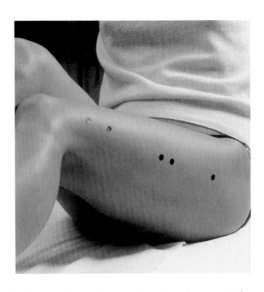

Illus. 35

In contrast to arthritis, (inflammation of the joints), arthrosis is the result of a prolonged, physically overtaxed bone structure that causes the deterioration of cartilage. Overweight, metabolic disturbances, and the normal aging process all contribute to the problem. If, in addition, poor circulation reduces the flow of appropriate nutrients to the bones, arthrosis is likely to develop.

Suggested treatment:

• Acupressure points: G 30, 31, 32, 33
• Corresponding magnet points: 77, 78, 79, 80, 81 special point

Attach five bio-magnets to the outside of the thigh—from the hip on down towards the knee as shown (G 30, 31, 32, 33) and an additional magnet to the "special point 81." Repeat this treatment often. Magnet foils and Yama magnets are also successful here.

Additional measures:

• Vitamins A and E, wheat germ oil and carrot juice
• Enzyme therapy
• Therapeutic baths, massage, sunbathing
• Drinking magnetized water
• Homeopathy: Kalium carbonicum D 3, Guajacum D 3, Cimifuga D 6, Calcium D 4

TRIGEMINAL NEURALGIA

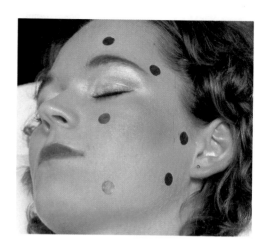

Illus. 36

Severe radiating pain, affecting only one half of the face, is usually a sign of this paroxysmal neuralgic disease of the cranial nerve. This nerve generates sensory stimuli to the head and face at the same time that it supplies motor activity to the jaws. Trigeminal neuralgia is much influenced by psychological stress, digestive disorders, colds, and exposure of the face to severe draughts. In all of these cases, start magnet therapy early.

Suggested treatment:

• Acupressure points: S 1, 3, 4, 8, TB 21, G 14
• Corresponding magnet points: 61, 69, 74, 66, 63

Apply bio-magnets to the most painful, sensitive points. Combining two methods is very useful: Several times a day move a Yama magnet, the white side to the skin, across the affected half of the face towards the ear. Supplement this by attaching small bio-magnets during the night, as shown. Repeat this treatment often.

Additional measures:

• Acupuncture therapy, in case of severe, prolonged pain
• Application of balm-spirit lotion
• Homeopathy: Aconit D 12, Magnesium phosphoricum D 4, Gelsemium D 6, Colocynthus D 4

GLAUCOMA

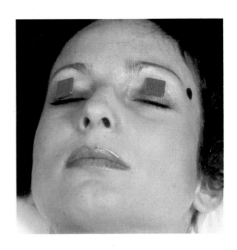

Illus. 37

Any sudden, severe pain in the eye, accompanied by disturbed vision and vomiting may be a sign of glaucoma. Immediate medical care is absolutely essential. Sustained or worsening eye pressure (intraocular pressure, which is part of the disease process) may damage the nervous system within the eye. Normal eye pressure is approximately 15. It is not unusual in cases of glaucoma for this pressure to go up as far as 70. This elevation of pressure in the eye is a malfunctioning of the central and the autonomic nervous system, which is interfering with the flow of fluids. Magnet therapy is an excellent adjunct to medical treatment.

Suggested treatment:

With eyes closed, attach one Marah-Cosam magnet (made in Switzerland from the very rare Samarium earth and cobalt), north (plus) pole to the skin, to the eyelid of the affected eye. This treatment should be done three times a day for fifteen minutes under medical supervision. Repeat it often.

Additional measures:

- Neck and shoulder massage
- Self-hypnosis/meditation
- Acupuncture therapy
- Vitamin B15
- Possibly fasting therapy
- Homeopathy: Ruta D 4, Atropinum sulfuricum D 6

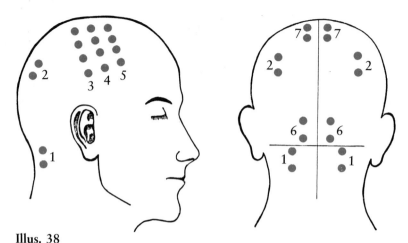

Illus. 38

The brain centers indicated above are often involved in specific illnesses. The numbers given them correspond to the conditions listed. Magnet therapy has proven beneficial when appropriately applied. It initiates a flow of energy and activates the centers in the brain so that they support the organism's own healing power.

Conditions appropriate to magnet therapy and their respective brain centers:
1. Impaired balance
2. Impaired speech
3. Painful extremities (arms and legs)
4. Paralysis
5. Treatment of tremors, chorea (Saint Vitus dance); athetosis (irregular, slow involuntary movements of fingers and toes); Parkinson's disease; apoplexy.
6. Vision problems
7. Problems in the sensory nervous system

Suggested treatment:

Using Yama magnets, massage the appropriate area with the white and black side several times a day for fifteen minutes each. Repeat this treatment often. Do not use magnet therapy in the presence of a brain tumor. Medical supervision is essential.

BURNS

The most common injuries in the home are burns, which can lead to severe disease symptoms. We distinguish between three different degrees of skin damage:

First degree: skin has turned red
Second degree: skin is blistering
Third degree: skin tissue has been damaged—medical treatment is essential.

First or second degree burns must be held under cold running water immediately to prevent blistering. Pain can be reduced quickly with the use of Yama magnets. But it is very important to disinfect the magnet with alcohol to prevent infections. Attach the Yama magnet (two, if needed), white side to the skin, to the burn site with a towel or bandage. The white side of the magnet has excellent bacteria-fighting properties so that the injury is able to heal without complications. If the burn site is small, the magnet can remain until the wound is healed. If the burn covers a larger area, consult a physician because of the danger of infection. Magnet therapy has shown excellent results in the follow-up treatment of painful scar tissue from burns. Scar tissue that has not healed properly or has become hard also reacts positively to treatment with magnets. Magnet foil, applied to the painful area where it increases blood circulation, results in a softening of the tissue with increased elasticity and elimination of pain.

Additional measures:

• Drinking magnetized water
• Vitamin A and E
• Homeopathy: Zincum metallicum D 8, Silicea D 12

PAINFUL SCARS

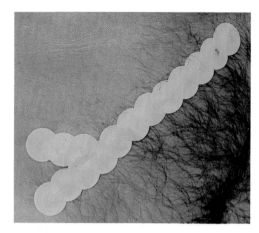

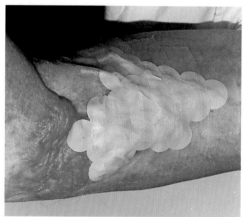

Illus. 40

Large, painful scars, such as from an operation, can lead to a disturbance of the energy flow, blocking the bioenergetic processes in the body. This disruption sends messages via the spinal cord to the brain where it registers as pain. In addition, scar tissue often becomes painful during changes in the weather.

Suggested treatment:

To re-establish an effective energy field around the scar, attach a bio-magnet or magnet foil to the scar tissue as shown in Illus. 39. Magnet therapy is also successful in the treatment of hypertrophic scar tissue and those that have grown into keloid tissue, as shown in Illus. 40. It has also been very effective in the treatment of chronic or acute infections of scar tissue. Repeat this treatment often.

Additional measures:

• Vitamin E
• Compresses with Comfry ointment
• Homeopathy: Graphit D 4, Silicea D 12, Zincum metallicum D 8

TOOTHACHE

In case of a toothache, only a trip to the dentist will bring relief—every sensible person knows that! But sometimes—as luck will have it—no dentist can be reached, often for days. In that case, don't reach for pain medications, because the chemical substances in them may be damaging to the liver and kidneys. Reach instead for a Yama magnet. The treatment is simple and will keep the pain in check until you can get an appointment. Pain after a tooth extraction may also be reduced by magnets. In case of swelling and when the roots have become infected, move a Yama magnet slowly across the painful area—white side touching the skin—three to five times daily for fifteen minutes. This treatment is also successful in case of receding gums—but here use the black side of the magnet to achieve a strengthening effect.

MUSCULAR PAIN

Painful muscles, either the result of over-exertion or of the harden-ing of the muscles, are a sign of a metabolic disturbance. Since the oxygen supply to the tissues during extreme muscle activity is insufficient, the conversion of glucose—the energy-spender—into oxygen is interrupted, and the remaining lactose accumulates in the tissues. When the substances needed for the breakdown of lactose are not available in sufficient quantities, metabolic residue accumulates. Not only does this residue cause pain, but it may also damage the muscular tissues.

Suggested treatment:

Locate the painful muscle zone and attach bio-magnets. The number of magnets will depend upon the size of the painful area. It is also possible to use magnet foil for this purpose.

Additional measures:

• Massage
• Electro-Acupuncture
• Therapeutic sulphur baths

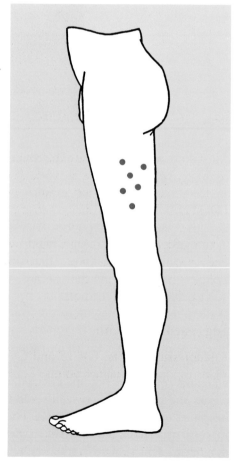

Illus. 41

STOMACH PROBLEMS
(Acute Gastritis)

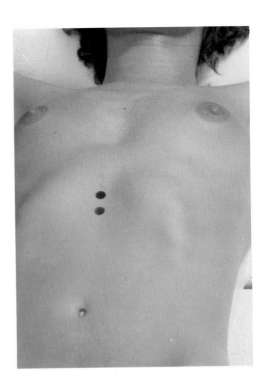

Illus. 42

Most stomach problems are the result of psychological stress, such as anger, worry, or stress at work. Food can literally "lie like lead in the stomach," causing cramps and discomfort. The diffuse pressure-like pain is usually accompanied by flatulence, lack of appetite, nausea, and diarrhea lasting a few hours or a few days. Acute gastritis is often aggravated by a poor diet high in acidity and by overindulgence in alcohol, nicotine, and coffee. The metabolic process is also affected, because it lacks the essential enzymes needed for proper digestion.

Suggested treatment:

- Acupressure points: CV 15 and CV 16
- Corresponding magnet points: 8 and 6

Below the sternum are two important pressure points that, when activated, have a calming influence on the stomach and help reduce discomfort. Attach bio-magnets to these pressure points, CV 15 + CV 16. Repeat this treatment often.

Additional measures:

- Enzyme therapy
- Drinking magnetized water
- Diet low in acidity
- Homeopathy: Antimonium crudum D 12, Arsenicum album D 6 to D 12, Colocynthis D 12, and in addition Aethiops antimonalis D 6

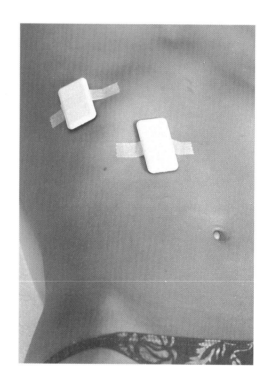

Illus. 43

Increased pressure from the fluid in the gallbladder causes a much dreaded intense pain. Often a by-product of anger and excitement, as well as the result of a rich diet high in fat, it makes itself known first by a "stuffed" feeling in the stomach area. It eventually produces cramps and nausea.

Suggested treatment:

• Acupressure points: Liv 14, 13
• Corresponding magnet point: 7, 9

As a first-aid measure Yama magnet therapy has been very effective. Attach two Yama magnets, black side touching the skin, above and below the rib cage as shown. Complement this with warm, moist compresses to reduce cramps and pain. If symptoms persist, X-rays and a medical examination are essential.

Additional measures:

• Drinking magnetized water
• Enzyme therapy
• Low-fat diet
• Homeopathy: Pulsatilla D 4, Lycopodium D 6, Flor de Piedra D 6

HEARING PROBLEMS (Tinnitus)

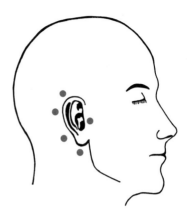

Illus. 44

Inner-ear hearing problems are often due to the aging process. The small nerve fiber of the inner ear becomes subject to hardening and subsequent shrinkage, which increases over time. The degree of hearing loss depends on the degree of the hardening process. Hearing ability, as a rule, will be bilateral, and high frequencies are the first to diminish. This type of hearing problem is called sound-sensory deafness. It is usually accompanied by a ringing of the ears.

Suggested treatment:

• Acupressure points: TB 17, 18, 19, 20, G 3
• Corresponding magnet points: 73, 71, 68, 65, 67

Attach four bio-magnets behind the ear, beginning with the first one directly in the indentation behind the ear lobe (TB 17). The last magnet is attached to the outside—at the entrance—of the ear canal, on the upper rim of the Arcus zygomaticus.

Additional measures:

• Neck massage
• Electro-acupuncture
• Vitamins A and E
• Homeopathy: Kalium chloratum D 4, Kalium jodatum D 2, Chininum sulfuricum D 3

80

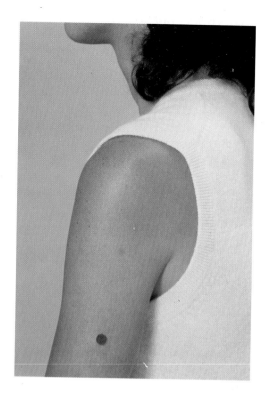

Illus. 45

The sensation of hunger is the downfall of all diets. So, if we want to lose weight we need to curb our appetite—to reduce the sensation of hunger. This is possible if we use our body's own "information network" to reach the hunger center in the brain.

Suggested treatment:

• Acupressure points: "yü-pe"
• Corresponding magnet point: 22

To lessen the sensation of hunger, attach one bio-magnet each at the midpoint on both upper arms. This point is located somewhat to the side, and it's easy to detect because the point is pressure sensitive. You'll notice the results in a couple of days, if you vibrate the magnet with gentle pressure several times a day. You can increase the effectiveness of this treatment by applying acupressure directly to a point located between the upper lip and the nose. Several times a day hold the skin at that point between your thumb and index finger, pressing gently for two minutes.

Additional measures:

- Scarsdale diet
- Helianthus tuberosus drops. They support detoxification and help reduce water retention. They are effective in treating metabolic disorders (also diabetes), gallstones, and other irregularities. Take ten drops four or five times a day, applied to the tongue. All of the above will reduce overweight.
- Enzyme therapy

4. Magnet-Foil Therapy

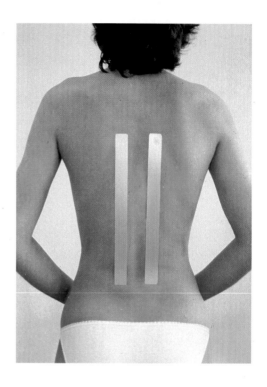

Illus. 46

Magnet foil is a variation of magnet therapy, in which ferromagnetic bio-magnets are applied to acupressure points. It is a simple procedure that is used when you need to cover a larger area than bio-magnets can. I came to it through my work in laser and acupuncture therapy, and used it for patients with "soft tissue" rheumatism. I observed in the course of the treatment that magnet foil, the same product that is used in industry, has definite therapeutic value. The patients reported a sensation of warmth in the field of application and a definite lessening of pain. This positive reaction is the result of the blocking of pain signals. It takes place when weak magnetic energy is applied to a biological unit of mass, energy, and metabolic processes as long as the pain stimuli is not too severe. Too high a dose of magnetic energy, as produced by electromagnetic fields, shows no positive results at all. It interferes with the resonating capacity of the body's cells as well as the fluctuating wave activity within each cell, which serves as an intercellular information process.

The function of pain is to signal the organism's distress to the cerebrum. The transmission of the message to the neurons in the brain, which is registering the situation, is—when viewed in terms of electricity—comparable to a flow of current: its strength is relative to the pain stimulus. The magnet foil at the pain site repolarizes the current and diminishes its flow. The result is a weakening of the energy load that is comparable to anesthesia. A shift in the ion-concentration at the cell membrane has taken place. Tests I conducted with magnet foil (with a strength of several hundred gauss) have shown positive results in treating the following conditions: muscle tension, back pain, rheumatism, and pain related to circulatory problems.

The therapy is relatively easy to use—even for a layperson. Cut a piece of magnet foil large enough to cover the painful area and attach it loosely—with skin-sensitive Band-Aids—to the body. Friction is created through the constant movement of the elasticized magnet foil against the skin resulting in magnetic alternate currents that relieve pain while they improve blood circulation and lessen tension. You can re-use the magnet foil repeatedly (see Illus. 46–48) until pain has disappeared and the organism has healed itself.

Treatment examples:

In case of pain and tension in the musculature of the back, attach two magnet foils, one left and one right of the spinal column.

In case of pain in the musculature of the shoulder and arm (soft-tissue rheumatism), cut the magnet foil to the desired size and attach to the pain area.

Magnet-foil therapy was also carried out successfully in cases of problems in the small pelvic area, the ovaries, fallopian tubes, and bladder, as well as uterine discharge. Medical supervision and follow-up examinations by a physician are imperative.

Illus. 47

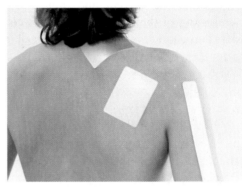

Illus. 48

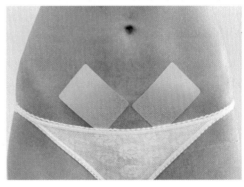

5. Acupressure Points and Magnet Points

On the pages that follow, you'll find charts of the human body on which we have indicated "magnet points," the key points on which to place bio-magnets or other magnets in order to treat the different problems that are listed below. These "magnet points" correspond to the acupressure points listed throughout the book. For example, the third eye, as stated on page 36, corresponds to magnet point 1; and acupressure point L I4 corresponds to magnet point 32 (see chart on page 89).

Ankles, pain in area of: 56, 57, 59, 83, 84, 85, 87

Asthma: 13, 19, 37, 38, 39, 40

Backache: 25, 26, 27, 28, 33, 84

Back and coccyx problems: 15, 28, 29, 30, 31, 84, 85

Bladder sensitivity: 11, 12, 15, 29, 30, 31, 58

Bronchitis: 5, 19, 37, 38, 39, 40

Cervical vertebra syndrome: 6, 17, 72

Circulatory problems: 16, 46, 59; connected with brain, 11, 16, 71, 72; connected with legs and feet, 15, 27, 28, 51, 55, 60, 82, 83

Colds: 5, 16, 17, 37, 38, 39, 40

Constipation: 7, 8, 9, 10, 11, 15, 30, 88

Cough: 13, 19, 37, 38, 39

Cystitis: 11, 12, 29, 30, 31

Depression: 6, 8, 14, 15, 42

Energy, lack of: 13, 42, 45, 55, 60

Eye Problems: 16, 32, 63, 64, 66, 86, 88

Fallopian tubes, problems with: 12, 29, 30, 84, 88

Flatulence: 7, 8, 9, 10, 11, 15, 27, 88

Gallbladder problems: 6, 7, 8, 15, 25

Hay fever: 32, 37, 38, 46, 64, 66, 70, 72

Headaches at the forehead: 1, 32, 61, 63, 66

Headaches at the back of the head: 16, 17

Headaches, *see Migraine*

Hearing problems: 65, 68, 69, 71, 72, 73

Heart, pounding: 4, 21, 40, 43, 46

Heart problems, nervous: 4, 19, 46

Hemorrhoids: 28, 29, 31

Hernia, problems in the area of: 27, 28, 52

High blood pressure: 14, 15, 46, 59, 75

Hip-joint problems: 28, 76, 77, 78, 79, 80, 81

Hoarseness: 2, 16, 38

Impotence: 29, 44, 45, 47, 52, 56

Insomnia: 1, 14, 15, 16, 46, 72, 88

Intestinal problems: 7, 8, 9, 10, 15, 25, 58

Kidney problems: 27, 28, 55, 60

Knee pain and arthrosis of the knee: 34, 48, 49, 50, 51, 53, 85, 88

Leg cramps: 35, 36, 54, 85, 88

Legs, heaviness: 28, 29, 53, 54, 55

Liver problems: 7, 9, 24

Lumbago: 25, 26, 27, 28, 84

Menopausal problems: 28, 29, 30, 31, 55, 67, 88

Menstruation problems: 12, 30, 31, 52, 55, 58, 67, 88

Migraine: 6, 7, 13, 16, 32, 55, 64, 67, 88

Nausea: 6, 7, 10, 16, 23, 46, 74

Neck problems: 16, 17, 32, 86

Nervousness: 5, 6, 8, 14, 15, 46, 88

Nicotine withdrawal: 14, 15, 16, 38, 46, 88

Nose problems: 1, 16, 64, 70

Nose, runny: 1, 16, 64, 70

Prostate gland problems: 29, 30, 31, 44, 45, 55

Sciatica: 25, 26, 27, 28, 33, 82

Shoulder pain: 17, 18, 19, 21, 23, 24, 84, 85

Shoulder problems: 17, 18, 19, 20, 21, 32

Sore throat: 2, 38

Stage fright: 6, 14, 15, 42, 46, 88

Stomach problems: 6, 8, 15, 23, 24, 25

Stomach ulcers: 6, 8, 10, 15, 88

Stress: 6, 7, 14, 15

Tennis elbow: 41, 42, 43

Test anxiety: 6, 14, 15, 42, 46

Travel sickness—dizziness: 6, 8, 14, 15, 73

Trigeminal neuralgia: 13, 32, 62, 63, 66, 69, 70, 74

Vision problems: 16, 63, 64, 66, 88

Weight loss: 6, 7, 9, 10, 12, 22, 55

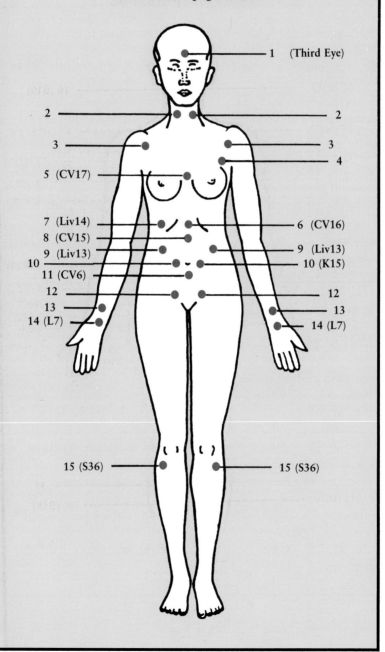

MAGNET POINTS 1–15
(and corresponding acupressure points)
referred to in pages 35–85

1 (Third Eye)

2

2

3

3

4

5 (CV17)

7 (Liv14)

6 (CV16)

8 (CV15)

9 (Liv13)

9 (Liv13)

10

10 (K15)

11 (CV6)

12

12

13

13

14 (L7)

14 (L7)

15 (S36)

15 (S36)

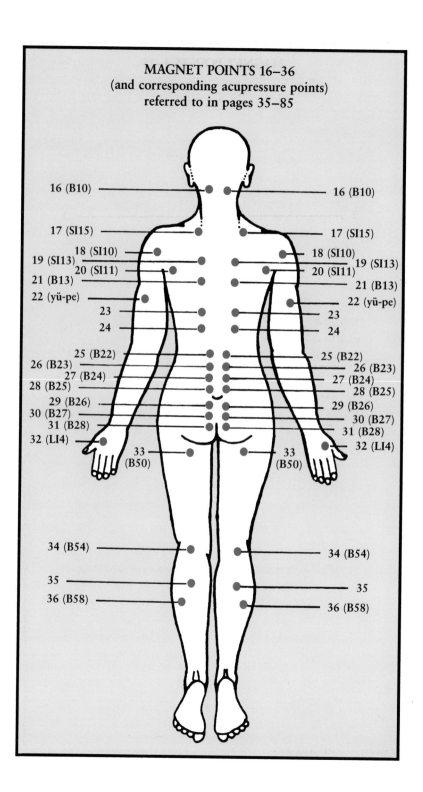

MAGNET POINTS 16–36
(and corresponding acupressure points)
referred to in pages 35–85

16 (B10)   16 (B10)
17 (SI15)   17 (SI15)
18 (SI10)   18 (SI10)
19 (SI13)   19 (SI13)
20 (SI11)   20 (SI11)
21 (B13)   21 (B13)
22 (yü-pe)   22 (yü-pe)
23   23
24   24
25 (B22)   25 (B22)
26 (B23)   26 (B23)
27 (B24)   27 (B24)
28 (B25)   28 (B25)
29 (B26)   29 (B26)
30 (B27)   30 (B27)
31 (B28)   31 (B28)
32 (LI4)   32 (LI4)
33 (B50)   33 (B50)
34 (B54)   34 (B54)
35   35
36 (B58)   36 (B58)

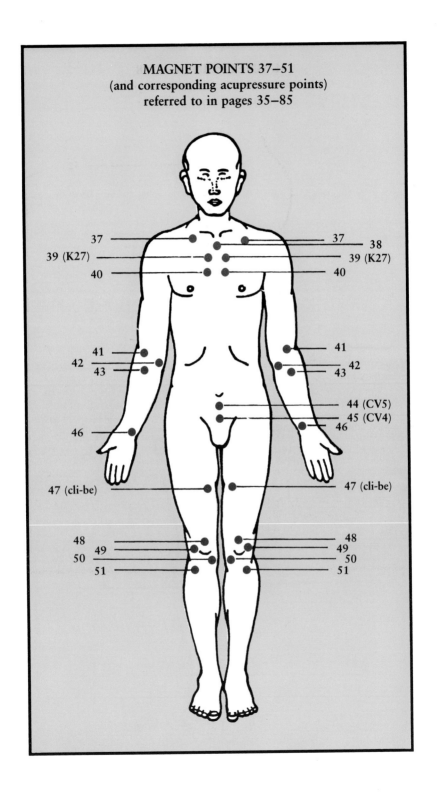

MAGNET POINTS 37–51
(and corresponding acupressure points)
referred to in pages 35–85

37   37   38
39 (K27)   39 (K27)
40   40

41   41
42   43   42
43   43

44 (CV5)
45 (CV4)
46   46

47 (cli-be)   47 (cli-be)

48   48
49   49
50   50
51   51

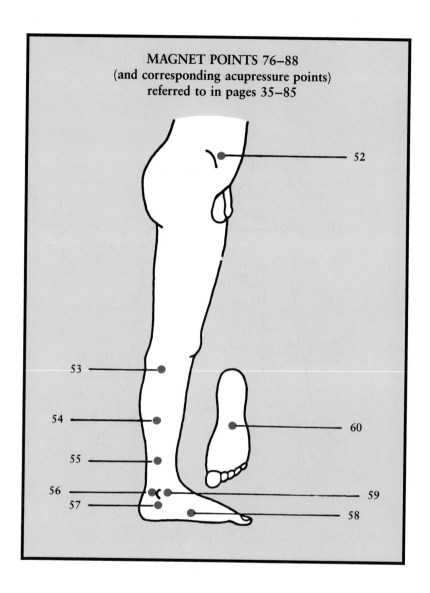

MAGNET POINTS 76–88
(and corresponding acupressure points)
referred to in pages 35–85

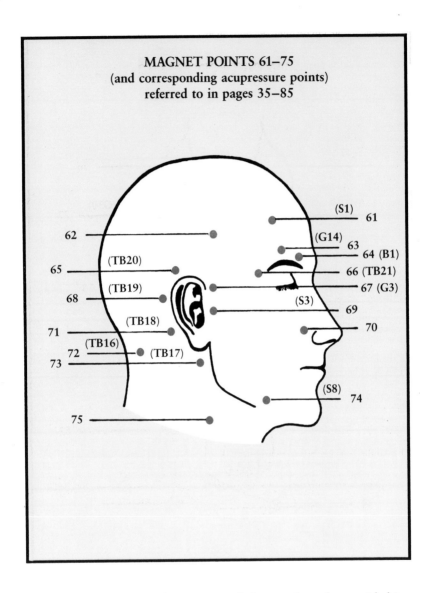

MAGNET POINTS 61–75
(and corresponding acupressure points)
referred to in pages 35–85

61 (S1)
62
63 (G14)
64 (B1)
65 (TB20)
66 (TB21)
67 (G3)
68 (TB19)
69 (S3)
70
71 (TB18)
72 (TB16)
73 (TB17)
74 (S8)
75

Professor Hannemann has requested that readers share with him successful treatments they have carried out using magnet therapy—if the treatments are not covered in this book. He would like to share these experiences and successful healing therapies with others who are seeking help. Please address all communications to him at Post Box 149, CH-9101 Herisau, Switzerland (fax 071/22 54 06).

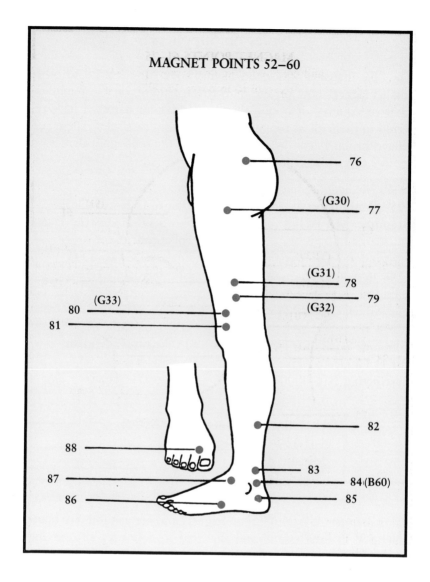

MAGNET POINTS 52–60

About the Author

Professor Holger Hannemann, M.Sc. practises magnet therapy in Herisau, Switzerland. In addition, he is a consultant and workshop leader dealing with this specialty. He has written several other books and articles about medicine.

Notes on Suppliers

The "bio-magnets" discussed in this book are identical to other small magnets now on the market. Depending on the manufacturer or country of origin, they have different names. I have referred to them all as bio-magnets, for neutrality's sake. These and related products can be purchased from the following sources:

OMS Medical Supplies, Inc.
1950 Washington St.
Braintree, MA 02184

Tools for Exploration
4286 Redwood Highway,
Suite C
San Rafael, CA 94903

Edmunds Scientific Co.
101 E. Gloucester Pike
Barrington, N.J. 08007

Intertrade Ltd.
Unit 6/11 North Close
Shorncliffe Industrial Estate
Folkestone, Kent
England, CT20 3UH
Fax (0303) 40 1 58

ITO Co., Ltd.
33 Toyotama-Minami
Nerima-Ku
Tokyo 176, Japan

Hisamitsu Pharmaceutical Co., Inc.
1-11-12 Minamisenba
Minami-Ku
Osaka, Japan

Yama magnets, Marah-Cosam magnets and magnet foils are manufactured in Switzerland and exported to countries all over the world. They come with detailed instructions in English. Write:

Naturheilpraxis
Post Box 149
CH-9101 Herisau
Switzerland

Index